"When it comes to managing PCOS symptoms, knowledge is power. For women with PCOS, Dr. Fiona McCulloch's groundbreaking new book is a wealth of this immediately applicable information that can make a difference in learning to manage their symptoms. Dr. McCulloch has interpreted all of the latest PCOS research and applied her own knowledge and expertise to create an easy-to-read, comprehensive resource. This brilliant book is the must-have guidebook for any woman who wants to manage her PCOS with a holistic lifestyle approach. Dr. Fiona can certainly be counted among the great PCOS medical experts, such as Dr. Walter Futterweit and Dr. Samuel Thatcher, who have blazed a trail of empowerment for the PCOS patient."

—**AMY MEDLING,** PCOS Diva

"Dr Fiona's eagerly awaited book on PCOS is everything I hoped it would be: comprehensive and insightful."

—**DR. LARA BRIDEN,** author, *The Period Repair Manual*

"*8 Steps to Reverse Your PCOS* is a detailed, engaging, and practical approach to the very complex issue of PCOS that it is easy to understand. Dr. Fiona puts each piece of the PCOS puzzle in place to provide a truly complete answer in restoring proper hormonal balance."

—**DR. MICHAEL T. MURRAY,** coauthor, *The Encyclopedia of Natural Medicine*

"I highly recommend this book! PCOS is a topic that is past due for global attention and clarity, and Dr. McCulloch's book delivers on these needs. *8 Steps to Reverse Your PCOS* helps readers understand if PCOS may be the hidden cause behind their weight gain, hair loss, or missed cycles. It will also help them understand why they are afflicted and give them a path back to health. The recommendations given are safe, well-balanced, and evidence-based, and they come from Dr. McCulloch's clinical experience and extensive research. The steps outlined also serve as an excellent guide for those with metabolic syndrome or prediabetes."

—**DR. ALAN CHRISTIANSON,** *New York Times* best-selling author of *The Adrenal Reset Diet*

"I was impressed by the comprehensive and integrative approach that Dr. McCulloch has achieved in this book, which will help women with this complex endocrinological disorder. Medicine's understanding of PCOS has come a long way in the last three decades, and Dr. McCulloch has grasped that evolution and embraced our modern scientific understanding of PCOS, including the science and importance of natural medicine in treatment strategies for PCOS"

—**DR. TORI HUDSON,** Clinical Professor, National University of Natural Medicine, Bastyr University, Southwest College of Natural Medicine; author, *Women's Encyclopedia of Natural Medicine*; Director of Education and Research, Vitanica; Medical Director, A Woman's Time

"Dr. McCulloch has done an impeccable job at capturing the whole picture of PCOS, including the emotional effects that are so commonly experienced throughout the journey. This book clearly and thoroughly outlines a step-by-step process that can be easily followed. *8 Steps to Reverse Your PCOS* is a must-have resource for women with PCOS, clinicians working with women's hormones or the emotional impact of having PCOS, and mothers of teenage daughters who may be experiencing symptoms related to PCOS. Knowledge is empowering, and Dr. McCulloch provides the knowledge and guides us through the actions necessary to grab hold of our life and turn it around!"

—**DR. JULIA SEN,** psychologist

8 Steps to Reverse Your PCOS

A Proven Program to Reset
Your Hormones, Repair Your Metabolism,
and Restore Your Fertility

DR. FIONA McCULLOCH, BSC, RAC, ND

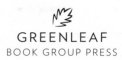

GREENLEAF
BOOK GROUP PRESS

This book is intended as a reference volume only, not as a medical manual. The information given here is designed to help you make informed decisions about your health. It is not intended as a substitute for any treatment that may have been prescribed by your doctor. If you suspect that you have a medical problem, you should seek competent medical help. You should not begin a new health regimen without first consulting a medical professional.

Published by Greenleaf Book Group Press
Austin, Texas
www.gbgpress.com

Copyright ©2016 Fiona McCulloch

Distributed by Greenleaf Book Group

For ordering information or special discounts for bulk purchases, please contact Greenleaf Book Group at PO Box 91869, Austin, TX 78709, 512.891.6100.

Design and composition by Greenleaf Book Group and Deborah Berne
Cover design by Greenleaf Book Group and Deborah Berne
Cover images: ©gettyimages.com/heroimages

Cataloging-in-Publication data is available.

Print ISBN: 978-1-62634-301-6

eBook ISBN: 978-1-62634-302-3

Part of the Tree Neutral® program, which offsets the number of trees consumed in the production and printing of this book by taking proactive steps, such as planting trees in direct proportion to the number of trees used: www.treeneutral.com

TreeNeutral®

Printed in the United States of America on acid-free paper

16 17 18 19 20 21   10 9 8 7 6 5 4 3 2 1

First Edition

To my husband, Shane—innovator and visionary—thank you for believing in me.

And to our sweet boys, Logan, Zachary, and Theo—you fill up my heart.

CONTENTS

FOREWORD

My first real introduction to polycystic ovary syndrome (PCOS) was in the nineties, early on in my acupuncture practice. While I had enough rudimentary information gleaned from the standard medical school curriculum, it merely touched upon how to diagnose this obscure and misunderstood "disorder" and medically control it, as there was no cure. The remedies at the time included the following:

1. Put the woman on oral contraceptives.
2. Treat her insulin resistance pharmaceutically (never mind the side effects).
3. Perform ovarian wedge surgical resection, if there were cysts.

Clomiphene was the only recommendation if infertility was part of the cascade. Rarely was this effective, and sometimes it worsened the presentation. There was no mention of dietary changes, modifying exercise, nutritional and supplement recommendations, or the effectiveness of acupuncture or herbs.

When my first atypical PCOS patient consulted me for help, I was at a loss. The Chinese medical literature did not address this scenario. I consulted other "experts" in the field of Oriental reproductive medicine, and none had success. There was nothing out there on treating this condition naturally. I scrambled. I researched, researched some more, and as my practice was getting busier, I started seeing the myriad presentations of different women who were diagnosed with PCOS. Some were thin. Some were heavy. Some had regular periods. Some had none. Some had other health conditions associated with their endocrine disorder that were being managed pharmaceutically. None were happy with their medical care. Each was trying to conceive.

A challenging environment presents itself for a pioneer in the field of natural reproductive medicine: You're on your own, and your laboratory is made up of patients who have no other options. You come to understand what the components of the health condition are. You apply different natural remedies (none proven). Some work. Some don't. Sometimes I could get patients who were not menstruating to menstruate, and the bleeding wouldn't stop! Then I'd have to try to control their bleeding before we could move on to encourage ovulation.

Months and years of trial and error gave rise to eventual success: The women who modified their diets, nutritional supplementation, and exercise regimens; took herbs; and received acupuncture were beginning to change. They no longer needed to take the troublesome drugs for insulin resistance and glucose intolerance. Their blood sugars were normalizing. Their periods become somewhat regular, and they started ovulating on their own. They even became pregnant.

While this approach was very effective, it wouldn't adhere to the medical criteria of double-blind, placebo-controlled, repeatable studies that would validate it with scientific research. Each woman had to be treated differently, based upon her unique presentation; thus, it was considered anecdotal.

PCOS is not a fixed diagnosis. It includes myriad presentations. It takes great dedication and interest in your patient to be able to find out what her unique cluster of systems consists of, and great patience, on both of your parts, to be able to find the remedy that will work for her.

Today the Internet abounds with information on natural care and PCOS management. Some work. Some do not. Much of my time has been spent conducting retreats and teaching Chinese medical professionals some of the nuances of natural reproductive care. I met Dr. Fiona McCulloch early on in my teaching career. She stood out among the rest of those working in her field. The first thing I noticed during one of our practitioner retreats was the depth of her empathy. She carried a profound wisdom that comes from having done her own healing work, which is unmistakable in a health-care professional: You naturally trust them, because you know they've been in the trenches and have come out better for it. They touch you in a place where the educated mind can't reach. She was honest, and she cared. The second thing I noticed about Dr. McCulloch was her uncanny knowledge. These are the types of people that you love having as students: the ones who *almost* know more than you do. They challenge you to stay on top of your game, because they are so sharp. As soon as she learned a new concept, she would master it, incorporate it into the wealth of knowledge she already had, and devour the next piece.

When Fiona asked me to evaluate her book, I couldn't wait. I was already beaming with pride and excitement. I sat down with her manuscript and was humbled. In fact, I was floored. There is nothing she hasn't covered. I went through her very detailed, easy-to-understand explanation of how to identify, address, and reverse PCOS. No longer do I consider her my student. Instead, she is *the* expert in the field of PCOS, whom I will consult when I encounter a challenging case.

There is nothing this book does not cover. Dr. McCulloch's easy-to-follow therapeutic guidelines are a must for anyone suffering from the effects of PCOS. The relationship with this condition has come a long, long way in just twenty-some years. If you have been diagnosed with PCOS, or if you carry the suspicion that you may have some of the symptoms of PCOS, start with this book. Learn to understand yourself first. Take charge of your own health and save yourself perhaps years of frustration in ineffective treatment cul-de-sacs. PCOS can be reversed. And Dr. McCulloch will show you how.

—Randine Lewis, PhD, L.Ac, author of *The Infertility Cure: The Ancient Chinese Wellness Program for Getting Pregnant and Having Healthy Babies* and *The Way of the Fertile Soul: Ten Ancient Chinese Secrets to Tap into a Woman's Creative Potential*

PREFACE

If you've just been diagnosed with polycystic ovary syndrome (PCOS), you might be feeling a great deal of confusion. You may be spending hours poring over Google to learn more about your condition and finding a lot that you relate with, but you are simply overwhelmed by the amount of information on PCOS. How do you know which of it applies to you?

Or perhaps you feel like the definitions and descriptions you are reading about don't describe your experience at all. Do you wonder why you don't exhibit the typical "textbook" presentation of PCOS (struggles with weight, facial hair, acne, and multiple cysts on your ovaries)?

Or you may suspect that you have PCOS, but nobody has formally diagnosed it, and doctors are puzzled by your case. Alternatively, you might have been diagnosed with the classic form of PCOS for many years and have tried a variety of treatments, but your symptoms just won't budge.

My hope is that this book will be a guiding light for you. It's my goal to give you more information about PCOS, to show you how to treat it effectively with natural medicine, and most of all, to empower you to understand your body.

As a young girl growing up in Toronto, I was always interested in health, science, and medicine. So, although I'm a naturopathic doctor now, it's in my nature to look at health through a scientific lens. My undergraduate science degree focused on cell and molecular biology, and I'm fascinated with the inner workings of our cells and the body's biochemistry.

When it comes to PCOS, I also have a personal story to tell. As a teenager, my periods started later than those of my friends. I was fifteen, nearly sixteen, years old. However, I was most unfortunately afflicted with cystic acne that made a grand entry all over my face before my periods even started. Once my cycles began, they were very irregular, as they were for many girls at that age. I remember learning in school that this was normal, and so I put it out of my mind.

For years, my periods continued on this way, coming with absolute randomness, but never any closer together than three months apart. There were many times that I would go six months without any sign of a period at all.

As a teenager, I was of average weight; however, I did gain fat around my middle and was heavier than I am currently. I overindulged in sugar and refined carbohydrates on a regular basis. I was always hungry and found it very hard to stop eating once I started. I was quite active, running long distances and playing racquet sports, so this probably kept my metabolism from going out of control.

Then I went to college and, like many of my friends, gained weight. My diet was composed mostly of sandwiches and the mountains of pasta they served regularly at the university cafeteria. Again, I tended to gain weight around my abdomen. I remember getting very sleepy after eating and finding it difficult to stay awake in class. At the time, I wasn't very in tune with my body and didn't give a lot of thought to my periods and their continued irregularity. Though I did continue to exercise and eat plenty of fruits and vegetables, it wasn't enough to override the effects of so many carbohydrates on my system.

In fact, at the time, I considered myself lucky that my periods didn't show up all that often—always referring back to the time in high school health class, when I learned that we were all unique and that it was normal if periods had very long spans between them. None of my friends, however, seemed to have the same sort of irregular cycles that I did.

My cystic acne raged on. While the skin of my friends began clearing up around age twenty, mine showed no sign of improving and, in fact, seemed to be getting worse. I traveled to Russia, doing a semester abroad, where at the time (1996) there were limited food options. There was, however, plenty of delicious, fresh bread, and this quickly became my staple. During my time there, I gained another ten pounds at my abdomen.

After returning home from Russia, I was at the point in my education where I needed to decide on a final path. I was torn. Should I become a research scientist or a medical doctor? I had always wanted to work in the field of medicine in some way. On visiting some laboratory environments, I realized that I really wanted to work with people, one-on-one, and I set my sights on medicine. In my last semester of college, I began to change my outlook on health. I joined the holistic health club, changed how I was eating, and visited a naturopath who helped me greatly.

I became intrigued with the new science that was burgeoning in the field of natural medicine and nutrition, given that my university was one of the leaders in research on nutrition in Canada. I was torn between traditional medical school and applying to naturopathic medical college. In the end, I decided that the route more true to my beliefs on health was to work with nutrition and natural medicine.

During my time at naturopathic medical school, I underwent a transformation. Armed with information on nutrition and diet, I lost the excess weight I had accumulated while in college. Immediately, my periods began to appear closer together, sometimes as close together as forty-five days. I wasn't sure what to attribute it to at the time. However, looking back, it's clear what caused this improvement.

What didn't improve was my cystic acne. It continued on, past graduation. Huge, painful, red pimples were constantly appearing on my jaw and chin, and they took months to fade away. I was desperate to clear up my skin. I had tried what seemed like everything available from dermatologists: long-term oral antibiotics like minocycline and tetracycline, tretinoin, topical antibiotics, and benzoyl peroxide. Many of these helped a little bit, but they were not getting at the underlying cause, and my acne persisted with a vengeance.

After graduation, I became interested in women's health and hormonal health and ran some hormone testing on myself. Considering all of my symptoms and signs, I was very curious to know if I had PCOS. In fact, my tests came back showing that I had a very high DHEA-S level, an androgen hormone often high in PCOS, and a reversed luteinizing hormone (LH) to follicle-stimulating hormone (FSH) ratio—two pituitary hormones that are often markers of PCOS. An ultrasound technician commented on how many follicles (eggs) I had in my ovaries. Everything made sense: the irregular cycles, the unrelenting acne that persisted well into my adult years. I also began experiencing the typical androgenetic alopecia (male-pattern hair loss) that is common in PCOS.

Once this information had been revealed, my doctor agreed with the diagnosis. I then began taking a variety of supplements and herbs, and my cycles shortened to twenty-eight days, where they remain. My body composition began to change, and the abdominal fat reduced. My acne improved considerably. Now I use a gentle essential oil formula as prevention. A pimple is a rare occurrence for me now and can almost always be attributed to something I've eaten. After many years of mainly anovulatory cycles, I had this major improvement in my hormonal health and was able to conceive three children, all boys, completely naturally. My last son was born when I was thirty-eight and, surprisingly, was the easiest for me to conceive.

I now have the tools that I need to keep my PCOS under control as I go through the next stages of my life. I know that although I am now forty-one years old, I still have a battle to face to keep my metabolism healthy, but I know exactly what to do and how to take care of myself.

Over the fifteen years of my clinical practice, I have seen improvements in my own hormones, and I've worked with many women with a variety of different conditions. I've focused on infertility, PCOS, thyroid disorders, and autoimmune disorders. Over time, I have realized that there is a strong interconnection between the hormonal systems, the brain, and the immune systems.

So, although many of the sections of this book may change as experts home in on the best criteria for diagnosing PCOS, what won't change is the need to look at and treat women with PCOS based on their unique biology. I am excited to share this information with you through this book—the product of many years of research, practice, and personal experience. My genuine hope is that it will empower you to improve your own health and well-being.

ACKNOWLEDGMENTS

First, I want to thank my patients. You have been my greatest teachers. From you, I have learned so much more than anything I could have ever read or researched. You've trusted me with your health, allowing me to gain insight into treating PCOS and other conditions, day after day, for the past fifteen years. I now offer up what I have learned from you in this book, in the hopes that it may help others.

Many thanks to those who helped me in making this book a reality. To Catherine W., thank you for editing my early versions of the manuscript, providing encouragement, and listening to more than one griping session with your typical grace. Thanks to my agent, Stephany Evans, who stuck by me patiently during the challenges of publishing a first-time author. Thanks to my dear friends Dr. Mary Wong, for late-night brainstorming sessions and mutual support, and Dr. Tanya Wylde, who shares my passion for this topic, for being a sounding board for ideas and research. Thank you to Dr. Randine Lewis for your ongoing mentorship and belief in me as an author, and to Dr. Michael Murray for your guidance and advice on my writitng journey.

To everyone at Greenleaf Book Group, thank you for your excellent teamwork and for making my dream of having this book published a reality. Thanks to my editors, Diana Ceres for your big-picture thinking and solid advice that transformed the structure of my material, and Lindsey Clark for your painstaking attention to detail and your patience. Gratitude to Debbie Berne for your phenomenal design work for my cover and layout.

Thank you to Dr. Erica Nikiforuk and Vee Zeniuk at White Lotus. You kept our patients well cared for while I wrote this book and held down the fort with strength and passion.

I also owe a lot to my parents, who came across the ocean from Scotland with just a trunk containing their belongings. They nurtured my curiosity and encouraged me with volumes of encyclopedias. They taught me to follow my passions and to never give up.

And finally, this book would not have been possible without my wonderful husband, Shane. You have fiercely encouraged me to keep writing, and your technical expertise always saves the day. Thank you for being the most dedicated partner in life and love and in raising our young family.

INTRODUCTION

A Guide to Using This Book

This book is designed as a step-by-step method to help you to address your PCOS. While the information presented is based on medical findings, it is intended to be an adjunct to your medical care, rather than a substitute. If you have been diagnosed with PCOS or think that you may have it, I encourage you to seek the medical assistance of your physician for routine care. The remedies presented in the chapters that follow, which are safe to take long term unless stated otherwise, may produce different results depending on your case, and as such, their use should always be supervised by your health-care practitioner. I urge you to follow up with your physician to monitor your condition, in case you need to adjust the dosage or remedy, depending on your unique situation.

The information in this chapter will show you how to use this book most effectively to manage your condition. After reading this chapter, take the quizzes at the end to determine if you have any of the traditional signs or symptoms of PCOS. Then you can proceed to the next chapter to learn more about PCOS, in case you are still wondering if you have the condition or need further information to make a determination. The remaining chapters provide guidelines on reversing your PCOS. At the end of the book, I have created some appendices that offer an array of information, ranging from fertility and pregnancy to menopause, prevention of diabetes and cardiovascular disease, and even some suggested recipes to help you manage and reverse your PCOS.

A Brief Overview of the Steps

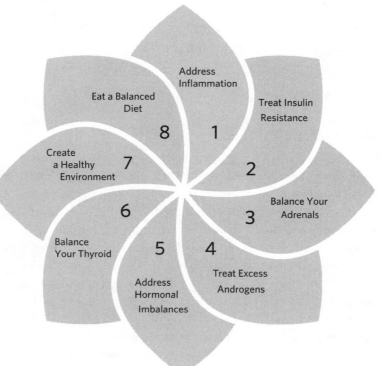

Inflammation

All women with PCOS should address inflammation, as this is the central underlying factor in PCOS according to current research. Women with a true autoimmune disease or other inflammatory conditions like type 2 diabetes should follow this even more closely. Take the inflammation quiz at the end of this chapter to determine how strongly you rate on this factor. Women who have a higher-than-average body mass index or gain weight around their abdomen will have markedly more inflammation, and a central part of improving inflammation will be following the nutrition recommendations in chapter 9.

Insulin Resistance

Most women with PCOS should address this factor, but women who have a waist circumference of more than thirty-five inches or who have struggled with their weight should place a lot of emphasis on this. You can take the insulin-resistance quiz to see how many signs of insulin resistance you have.

Some women with PCOS, particularly those who are very lean, may have very minimal or undetectable insulin resistance. For these women, following a strict diet will not provide the same results that you would see in women who have significant insulin resistance. Instead, the nutrition recommendations should be considered, but more focus must be placed on the hormonal and inflammatory aspects. It's important to remember that even in women who do not have detectable insulin resistance, the ovaries are sensitive to excesses of insulin compared to women without PCOS.

Adrenals, Stress, and Mood

Women with PCOS should take the adrenals quiz before addressing this factor. For most women with this condition, the adrenals and stress will be involved to some degree. This is particularly the case for women who have adrenal androgen excess PCOS. Just like the ovary, the adrenal glands, which are situated on top of the kidneys, can produce androgenic hormones. This is almost a unique type of PCOS that can be different in a variety of ways. I've found that many lean women with PCOS have adrenal androgen excess, as adrenal androgens do provide a degree of protection against the metabolic sluggishness that is often seen in PCOS.

Androgen Excess

Most women with PCOS will need to address this factor. For women who don't have any points on the androgen quiz, androgen excess is still usually present in small amounts within the tissue of the ovaries and can actually be reduced by working on insulin resistance, pituitary-ovary regulation, and inflammation. Androgen excess is one of the central factors in PCOS. High androgens within our ovaries can stall ovulation, and too many androgens in our skin cause unwanted hair growth, hair loss, and acne. As you'll read in the chapter on androgen excess, you'll need to become a detective to determine if you have this factor, as blood tests can be misleading.

Hormonal Imbalances

Women with PCOS should take the quiz related to this section before addressing this factor. Although androgen excess is one of the major hormonal challenges you'll see in PCOS, there's often dysregulation of hormones, such as estrogen and progesterone, as well as the pituitary hormones LH and FSH. Not all women with PCOS have problems with ovulation, although most do at some point in their lives. Having good balance and positive feedback between the hormones of the ovary (estrogen and progesterone) and the hormones of the brain and pituitary (LH and FSH) is the key to feeling your best, preventing mood disorders, and having regular menstrual cycles. That being said, in many women, by the time the prior factors, such as inflammation and insulin resistance, are worked on, these other hormonal imbalances may have resolved. And some women may have very little insulin resistance but a lot more imbalance within their pituitary-ovary hormones. So this is why we always have to treat patients as individuals, looking for which factors are strongest on a case-by-case basis.

Thyroid

Women with PCOS should take the thyroid quiz before addressing this factor. It is a major aggravating factor but isn't present in all women with PCOS. Thyroid disease, such as autoimmune thyroiditis, is more common in women with PCOS. Since a low-functioning thyroid makes insulin resistance worse, and insulin resistance makes thyroid function lower, this is very important to look for and address in any woman with PCOS. Studies have even found that there may be special PCOS-specific ranges for thyroid function that are different from the usual, so you'll want to become educated on this before you get bloodwork done.

Environment

The environment has a profound effect on women's health. It's been found that the effects of environment persist for generations, passing down hormonal issues to our children and grandchildren. Many toxins exist that affect the presentation and severity of PCOS, including those found in plastics like BPA, dioxins, and pesticides. All women should read the suggestions in this chapter and try to incorporate them into their lives, but those who score highest on the quiz may be impacted more by environmental concerns and should pay special attention to chapter 8, which outlines how to cultivate a more healthy environment.

Diet and Nutrition

It goes without saying that one of the most important factors for women with PCOS is a healthy diet. PCOS is probably the women's health condition that responds the best to dietary changes. In some cases, nutrition alone can reverse most symptoms. Since most women with PCOS suffer from at least some degree of insulin resistance, and all have inflammation, following an anti-inflammatory nutrition plan that regulates insulin levels is often the best approach. That being said, the nutritional approach for a lean woman with PCOS is different from that for a woman with a higher body mass index. There are also a variety of different diets that can provide successful results. Furthermore, there are some women who already follow an excellent nutrition plan but still suffer from symptoms. This goes to show that PCOS is a truly diverse condition—one that is unique to each and every woman.

Quizzes

The following quizzes will help pinpoint your symptoms to determine which factors are most important to treat in your presentation of PCOS. Take a moment to take each quiz to see where you lie in the PCOS spectrum. If you test strongly for particular areas, you will want to pay close attention to the chapters that correspond to these symptoms in this book. If you're not sure if you have PCOS, see the quizzes included in chapter 1 to help determine if you do.

Inflammation Quiz

Inflammation is a key factor. All women with PCOS have it. As you'll see below, you will either have moderate or severe inflammation.

1. I have pain in my body, such as neck pain, back pain, knee pain, or headaches.
2. I have skin rashes, such as eczema, psoriasis, rosacea, or allergic dermatitis.
3. I have chronic digestive problems, such as bloating, diarrhea, ulcers, reflux, or indigestion.
4. I have asthma or allergies.
5. I'm constantly tired and lethargic.
6. I eat a diet that is not based on whole foods and contains many processed foods and sugars.
7. I have a family member with an autoimmune disease.
8. I have been formally diagnosed with PCOS.

If you have answered yes to five to eight of these, it's likely you have severe inflammation. If you've answered yes to one to four of these, it's likely you have moderate inflammation.

Insulin Resistance Quiz

1. My waist is thirty-five inches or more, if I'm normal to large framed, or thirty-two inches or more if I'm small framed.
2. I gain weight predominantly around my abdomen.

3. I crave sugar.

4. I have struggled with weight loss.

5. I crave carbohydrates, such as rice, bread, and potatoes.

6. I don't feel full easily and eat too much at one sitting, or I binge at times.

7. There are people in my immediate family who have diabetes (mother, father, grandparents, siblings, aunts/uncles).

8. I am sensitive to not eating for periods of time and experience symptoms of hypoglycemia, such as shakiness, irritability, or dizziness.

9. I have dark, velvety patches in the folds of my skin behind my neck, at the crease of my thighs, or under my arms (acanthosis nigricans).

10. I have skin tags.

11. I have a fatty liver.

If you have answered yes to seven to eleven of these, it's likely you have severe insulin resistance. If you have answered yes to three to six of these, it's likely you have moderate insulin resistance. If you've answered yes to zero to two of these, you may have mild or undetectable insulin resistance.

Adrenals and Stress Quiz

1. I have a lot of stress in my life.

2. I have experienced extreme stress in the past five to eight years.

3. I do not get enough sleep.

4. I have anxiety.

5. I have depression.

6. I consume too much sugar.

7. I have heart palpitations.

8. I drink a lot of coffee to get through the day.

9. I get irritated easily.

10. I have serious mood symptoms when I have PMS.

11. I have low blood pressure.

12. I have dizziness when I stand up too quickly.

13. I overwork and do not take time to relax.

14. I have taken steroids for a medical reason.

15. I gain weight around my abdominal area.

16. I have an eating disorder now or have had one in the past (binge eating, anorexia, bulimia, or orthorexia).

17. I have a low libido.

18. My muscles feel weak.

19. I feel very tired between 3:00 and 5:00 p.m.

20. I feel best in the evening.

21. I have had high DHEA-S readings on bloodwork.

If you have answered yes to fourteen to twenty-one of these, it's likely you have a severe adrenal/stress factor. If you have answered yes to five to thirteen of these, it's likely you have a moderate adrenal/stress factor. If you've answered yes to one to four of these, it's likely you have a mild adrenal/stress factor.

Androgen Excess Quiz

1. I have hirsutism: the growth of excess or coarse hairs on my chin, face, upper lip, chest, or abdomen.

2. I have significant acne that is present after the age of twenty. The acne is concentrated around the jawline, back, or chin or has recurred after intensive treatment, such as isotretinoin or birth control pills.

3. I have hair loss that is either diffuse or is concentrated behind the front hairline.

4. I have a deep voice.

5. I have high DHEA-S, testosterone, androstenedione, or DHT levels on blood testing.

If you have answered yes to *any* of these, you have the androgen excess factor to a significant degree.

Hormone Balance Quiz

1. My cycles are or have been thirty-five days or longer for significant periods of time in my life.

2. I've had polycystic ovaries on ultrasound.

3. I ovulate late in my cycle—around day eighteen or later.

4. I've needed to take medications to help me ovulate.

5. The medications intended to help me ovulate didn't work on at least one occasion.

6. I've had a high anti-Mullerian hormone (AMH) reading on a blood test.

7. I've had a high luteinizing hormone (LH) to follicle-stimulating hormone (FSH) ratio on a day-three blood test.

8. I have had low progesterone readings on bloodwork.

If you have answered yes to *any* of these, you have the hormonal imbalance factor to a significant degree.

Thyroid Quiz

1. I feel cold compared to others around me.

2. I feel tired a lot or exhausted without reason.

3. I do not lose weight easily, despite dieting and exercising.

4. I am constipated.

5. I have dry, flaky skin.

6. I'm losing hair: It is brittle, coarse, and dry. Or, I am losing outer eyebrow hair.

7. My nails are brittle.

8. I'm depressed or anxious.

9. I have chronic muscle and joint pains.

10. I feel pressure or swelling in my neck, have difficulty swallowing, and my voice has become hoarse.

11. I have a family member with thyroid disease or an autoimmune disease.

12. I have high cholesterol that does not respond to diet changes or medication.

13. I have unexplained changes in my weight, unrelated to my lifestyle.

14. I have changes in my memory and concentration.

15. I have had abnormal thyroid testing results (including autoimmune thyroid antibody testing) or am taking thyroid medication already.

If you have answered yes either to number fifteen alone, or to ten to fifteen of these, you have a significant thyroid factor. If you haven't been tested, you should be. If you have answered yes to five to nine of these, you have signs of a moderate thyroid factor and lab testing is warranted. If you have answered yes to one to four of these, you have some signs of a thyroid factor and lab testing is warranted.

Even if you are taking thyroid medication and your condition is under control, I still recommend reading through the thyroid chapter so that you can optimize your thyroid health with nutrition and lifestyle. The thyroid is complex, and medication often only approximates what our thyroid function would be naturally.

Environmental Factors Quiz

1. I do use, or have in the past used, plastic containers to a significant degree for reheating food, or I have used plastic water bottles.
2. I do currently eat, or have eaten, canned foods, including soda from cans.
3. I was fed from a plastic baby bottle or plastic sippy cups as an infant.
4. I have worked in retail, handling receipts.
5. I work in the dental profession, a hair/nail salon, or other profession where I am exposed to environmental toxins.
6. I buy primarily nonorganic produce, dairy, or meats.
7. I have worked in agriculture or gardening with pesticides, or my mother was exposed to pesticides prior to being pregnant with me.

If you have answered yes to one to three of these, you have a moderate environmental toxicity factor. If you have answered yes to four to seven of these, you have a significant environmental toxicity factor.

All women with PCOS should address the environmental toxicity factor, as it is impossible to escape these pervasive effects on health. Although we can't fully protect ourselves or future generations from toxicity, there are some ways we can reduce the impacts.

Diet and Nutrition Quiz

1. When I have made changes in my diet in the past, I've seen significant improvements in my PCOS symptoms.
2. There are areas of my diet that I feel could use some improvement.
3. I consume fast food or sweets at least twice per week.
4. I have intense cravings for sugar or carbohydrates.
5. I find it difficult to stop eating, or I binge at times.
6. I don't get enough vegetables in my diet.
7. I'm not really sure what I should be eating.

8. I know what to do with my diet, but I find it hard to actually make good decisions when the time comes to eat.

9. I tend to eat the same foods all of the time.

10. I go through periods of eating well, followed by periods of eating poorly.

11. I scored moderate to high on the insulin resistance quiz (three to ten yes responses).

If you have answered yes to one to four of these, you have a moderately high need for nutritional support and would benefit from making dietary changes. If you have answered yes to five or more, you would benefit significantly from making nutritional and dietary changes.

Your Factors

First, complete the table below by circling the factors you have and their intensity in your case. Then read through each chapter of the book. Work on the factors that you have, to the degree warranted by your rating on the quiz. For example, if you have significant insulin resistance, you would want to read that chapter carefully and follow the recommendations closely. If, conversely, you don't have a lot of female hormonal imbalance and you ovulate regularly, you may benefit more from the content in other chapters.

Table I-1 lists each of the eight key factors. Please circle your individual level of significance for each factor that you calculated in the quiz. You can refer to this later as you work through each chapter in the book.

FACTOR	YOUR INDIVIDUAL LEVEL OF SIGNIFICANCE		
Inflammation		Moderate	Significant
Insulin Resistance	Mild/Undetectable	Moderate	Significant
Androgen Excess		No	Yes
Hormone Balance/ Ovulation		No	Yes
Adrenal	Mild	Moderate	Significant
Thyroid	Mild	Moderate	Significant
Environment	Mild	Moderate	Significant
Nutrition and Diet	None	Moderate	Significant

You may need to spend more time on one step, particularly if you have a signifi-cant factor in that area, whereas you may not need to spend as much time with other steps. Another consideration is that when you work on the underlying causes, like inflammation and insulin resistance, you may see problems resolve in some of the other areas before you get there, and you may not need to work on those areas at all.

All women should implement environmental measures throughout their pro-cess, regardless. The sooner you can make changes to improve your environment the better, particularly for those women who are trying to conceive, as it's been found that environmental factors can affect future generations.

This book is detailed and is meant to include most of the information we cur-rently know about PCOS. If you'd like to follow me on my blog or on Facebook, I regularly share the basic concepts that are introduced here, and in time they will become familiar to you. I've found my patients want the most comprehensive infor-mation on PCOS, and so I've included all of the information here, so you can go through it as time permits—though understanding every detail is not required to improve your health. Always feel free to reach out to me via my blog or through social media if you are interested in learning more about any of the concepts I've illustrated in the book.

Chapter 1

DEFINING PCOS

*To be yourself in a world that is constantly trying to make
you something else is the greatest accomplishment.*
—RALPH WALDO EMERSON

Sophia leaned forward at the restaurant table toward her friend Elizabeth, as if she were hearing an intensely fascinating secret. Sophia and Elizabeth met last year at the marketing company they worked for and had more recently been developing a friendship. Sophia's slim arm rested on the tabletop, her eyes unable to conceal their surprise and interest. She was a tall, lean woman, with a tendency to anxiety.

Elizabeth was far curvier than her friend, with glowing, clear skin. Elizabeth struggled with what she called her "apple shape," carrying a lot of weight around her belly, despite the many diet programs she had embarked on over the years.

"So, you have it too?" Elizabeth spoke to her friend in a hushed tone, looking sideways, as if ensuring that nobody was listening to their conversation.

"I do." Sophia gestured to her jawline, which was inflamed with angry-looking pimples. "You'd think I'd be past this stage by age thirty-four!"

As a young woman of thirteen, Sophia's period began as expected. Around the same time, her skin began to break out terribly, particularly along her jawline and on her back. Her periods were always irregular, arriving at their leisure (usually about two months apart), bringing with them intense cramps and heavy bleeding. Over time, Sophia developed coarse hair on her chin and cheeks. This was a great source of distress. She spent many hours trying different hair-removal techniques and attempting to find treatments for her acne, none of which were particularly effective.

Last year, after doing some online research, Sophia asked to be referred to a gynecologist, and her bloodwork came back with high levels of testosterone. The doctor diagnosed her with PCOS: polycystic ovary syndrome.

Once home, Sophia immediately Googled PCOS, intent on finding out more about the condition that had caused her so much difficulty. What she found was a great deal of confusing information. Descriptions of voluptuous women with ovarian cysts and high testosterone levels seemed to be central to almost every article on the topic. Much of it didn't match Sophia, as her ultrasound did not show any cysts, and she was a very slim woman. She knew that her testosterone was high, but she wondered why her case was so different from most of the other women who had the same diagnosis.

Elizabeth, on the other hand, had been diagnosed with PCOS at a young age. As a child, she had always struggled with her weight, and as she reached adolescence, she began gaining weight quickly. Both her mother and sister had a similar body composition, as did many of her extended female relatives. As a teenage girl, Elizabeth was elated to get her first period, but it did not return again for another ten months. Although many of her friends experienced a similar irregularity at first, eventually their periods became regular. It was not so for Elizabeth. This was how her cycles continued on: She averaged two periods per year. She dreamed of having normal cycles and feeling feminine like her friends, but her cycles never regulated on their own. Unfortunately, Elizabeth usually had to take a course of prescription medication to bring on her monthly menstruation.

Elizabeth had many ultrasounds of her ovaries over the years, and they were always full of small, round cysts—the classic "string of pearls" described in textbooks. Similarly to Sophia, Elizabeth also had hair growth on her chin and cheeks, but it was blond and fine, and most people didn't really notice it.

Elizabeth had married a wonderful man when she was thirty-two, and they desperately wanted to start a family together. Again, things weren't easy: Together, they began an intense battle with infertility that had been going on for the past two years. The fertility clinic felt like a second job to her. It was an extra place she had to go each morning, bright and early at 7:00 a.m., something she despised.

She felt consumed by the "project" of getting pregnant: charting, peeing on sticks, waiting and agonizing for two weeks every month, along with medications, stirrups, ultrasounds, and procedures. When it didn't work, which was always, she had to do it all over again the following month. Why couldn't she just conceive easily, like all of her friends did?

"So, you have PCOS, too? I'm surprised! It's just that you just don't look like . . . " Elizabeth trailed off, taking a sip of her sparkling water, feeling a sense of hesitant camaraderie.

"I do, though I find my case isn't the 'typical' sort," Sophia replied. "One thing I do know is that whatever it is that I have going on with my hormones, it's definitely causing me a lot of grief."

How could these two very different women have the same syndrome?

A Brief History of PCOS: A Disorder with Many Faces

Do you ever wonder why PCOS has so much variability? More and more information on PCOS is being revealed at a rapid pace, with hundreds of new studies released each year.

PCOS has long been a mystery in women's health, as the underlying causes were never fully understood. Back in 1935, two researchers, Stein and Leventhal, described a group of larger-sized women that had coarse, male-pattern hair growth (known as hirsutism) on their faces. This group also had enlarged ovaries with multiple small cysts and irregular menstrual cycles. They named the condition Stein-Leventhal syndrome. Since that time, the diagnosis has expanded and includes many women far outside of the typical sort of PCOS that they had initially described.

The information, types, and definitions of PCOS used in this book are based on current research and on my clinical experience in treating hundreds of women with the condition. As the research grows, many of the concepts in this book may be expanded upon or entirely changed. The understanding of PCOS is really just beginning, and I look forward to seeing it grow.

Interestingly, there is a movement to change the name of PCOS from polycystic ovary syndrome, as many women with the syndrome do not actually have polycystic ovaries at all. The new name is still being debated but is hoped to express the many different types of the condition.

As the most common hormonal disorder in women of reproductive age, PCOS affects an estimated 116 million women worldwide and can affect hormones, fertility, the skin, cardiovascular health, and metabolism. PCOS is called a syndrome, rather than a disease, as there is a wide range of ways that PCOS can present and a variety of factors that characterize it.

PCOS can be expressed in women with excessive androgenic hormones like testosterone, producing acne and hair growth as we've seen in Sophia's case. Or it can present similarly to Elizabeth, with abdominal weight gain, infertility, and loss of ovulation and menstrual cycles.

This is why researchers have been puzzled about PCOS for years, with significant argument between professional groups about what constitutes a diagnosis of PCOS. In the last decade, however, there has been some agreement that there are, in fact, different "types" or phenotypes of the disease, which explains why two women with PCOS might look very different.

In 1990, the National Institute of Health (NIH), one of the world's foremost medical research centers, defined PCOS as requiring three criteria:

1. Delayed ovulation or periods, known as oligoovulation

2. Excess androgens, such as testosterone or DHEA, causing acne,

hirsutism, male-pattern hair loss, or high androgens on a woman's
bloodwork

3. Other conditions that would create a similar syndrome would have to
    be excluded

Interestingly, the NIH did not require a woman to have ovarian cysts to receive
a diagnosis of PCOS. Overall, the NIH criteria are stricter, and fewer women have
PCOS according to this definition.

Rotterdam and the Three Criteria

In 2003, there was a meeting in Rotterdam, the Netherlands, sponsored by two of
the top reproductive medicine groups: one European (ESHRE) and one American
(ASRM). Together, leading experts gathered in this northern city to focus on refin-
ing the definition of PCOS. The meeting produced what are known as the Rotterdam
criteria, which are arguably the most widely accepted criteria for the diagnosis of
PCOS.[1]

This meeting produced something else that caused quite a stir in the world of
endocrinology. What made the Rotterdam criteria different in diagnosing PCOS was
that women didn't need to have all three of the characteristics. **Only two of the three
were required for a diagnosis.** This gave birth to the idea of different phenotypes or
"PCOS Types." It also produced two totally new "types" of PCOS, which didn't exist
before.

The three criteria introduced by the Rotterdam consensus were—

1. Delayed ovulation or menstrual cycles (anovulation)
2. Hyperandrogenism/high androgenic hormones like testosterone
3. Polycystic ovaries on ultrasound

It's important to note that PCOS is a very complex disorder, and that these types
are mainly a holding place for what we understand as of now. These types will likely
change over time as we learn more about what makes up this complex and common
condition in women's health.

Symptoms of PCOS

PCOS has myriad symptoms, ranging from hair loss to fatigue and weight gain.
These various symptoms fall into three main categories, as evidenced by the Rotterdam consensus. For a woman to be diagnosed with PCOS, she must exhibit two of
the three required criteria (anovulation, hyperandrogenism, and polycystic ovaries).
Let's take a moment to explore each of the criteria in more detail.

Anovulation

Anovulation translates as "lack of ovulation," but in medical terms, it can also mean ovulations that are delayed past the typical timing. The average length of a woman's menstrual cycle is twenty-eight days. Day one of the cycle is the first day of the period, and most women will ovulate on or around day fourteen, give or take a few days.

Anovulation is technically defined as *fewer than ten menstrual cycles per year*. This would be equal to having menstrual cycles thirty-five days or longer in length. If you'd like to know more about menstrual cycles, please see chapter 6 for a comprehensive explanation of how the hormones, ovulation, and menstrual cycles work in PCOS.

Anovulation

- Fewer than ten menstrual cycles per year

   OR

- Cycles that are thirty-five days long or longer

As you can see, if you have regular menstrual cycles, but they are longer than average, you may still have anovulation. This is something I see often in practice: longer-than-average cycles, though they may appear regularly. Many women actually believe this is a normal thing, but it's most definitely not. Cycles that are thirty-five days in length or longer (even if they are regular) are a red flag for PCOS, particularly if a woman's cycle has been longer since her teenage years.

As women age, their cycles often naturally become shorter, so anovulation may be resolved by Mother Nature as a woman matures. That said, if a woman had long cycles for many years when she was younger, as well as the other characteristics of PCOS, it is a sign that she should be assessed more closely.

Hyperandrogenism

Hyperandrogenism is a very long word that basically means there are high levels of hormones, such as testosterone, DHEA, or androstenedione. These particular hormones are responsible for causing male sexual characteristics like the growth of facial and body hair and hair loss in specific patterns.

Symptoms of Hyperandrogenism

- Hirsutism: hair growth on the chin, upper lip, around the nipples, on the chest or stomach, on the upper arm or thigh, or in other areas
- Acne, particularly along the jawline or on the back (Androgenic acne is often moderate to severe.)
- Hair loss in an androgenic pattern; frontal with hairline preserved or diffuse
- Elevated hormones like testosterone, DHEA, or androstenedione

In chapter 5, there will be a comprehensive discussion with more details on these symptoms.

PCOS "Cysts"

At Rotterdam, researchers went through what it means to have polycystic ovaries. They determined that there must be twelve or more follicles measuring from two to nine millimeters or an ovarian volume bigger than ten centimeters in a single ovary. Follicles are the spherical structures in the ovary that house the eggs. On ultrasound, many women with PCOS have a larger than average number of follicles. Even if only one ovary shows an excess number of follicles or "cysts," this can be suggestive of PCOS.

If you request an ultrasound, you can ask the technician to include the ovarian volume and to look at the number of smaller follicles in your ovary and to count them. It's often best to have this ultrasound done on the third day of your menstrual bleed, but if you're not having menstrual cycles regularly, you can also have this done on any given day. In women who don't menstruate often, there is an increased chance of seeing these types of follicles regardless of the cycle day.

PCOS "Cysts" Include—

- Twelve or more follicles ranging from two to nine millimeters in a single ovary
- Ovarian volume bigger than ten centimeters in a single ovary
- With newer ultrasound technology, more than twenty-six follicles that are two to nine millimeters in both ovaries

Now, let's talk about the cysts in the ovary and what they actually are. They are not true ovarian cysts, like those found in women without PCOS. One of the most common types of non-PCOS cysts is the simple functional cyst: these are large, fluid-filled sacs within the ovary that resolve on their own and happen in many women occasionally. Another type of non-PCOS cyst is the "complex" ovarian cyst: These are larger cysts that contain a variety of different types of cells and may contain blood or other tissues. In most cases, the number of simple or complex cysts is far lower than the number of "cysts" found in a woman with PCOS (often only one cyst is present, or just a few).

PCOS cysts are in fact different from both of these and are not even true cysts at all! So why do some women with PCOS have so many follicles on ultrasound? In a healthy ovary, the follicles go through a slow state of growth known as folliculogenesis for many months before the egg is ready to be ovulated.

In PCOS, this process can become stalled because of high testosterone and insulin in the ovary. The outer layer of the follicle known as the theca, which produces testosterone, thickens, and the follicles stall in their development process and accumulate in the ovaries rather than going through ovulation.

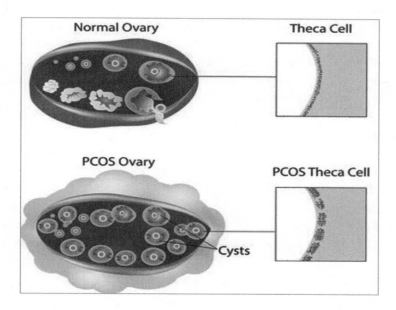

Figure 1-1: PCOS "Cysts." Cystic appearance of the ovary in PCOS versus a typical ovary. Note the thickening of the theca layer of the follicles. Courtesy of the National Institutes of Health: Eunice Kennedy Shriver National Institute of Child Health and Human Development.

As such, PCOS "cysts" are actually just ovarian follicles that are in a state of partial development. Over time, these partially developed follicles pile up in the ovary, creating the look of multiple tiny cysts, or what is often referred to in textbooks as a "bunch of grapes" or a "string of pearls."

PCOS Cysts and Age

Ovaries with multiple small follicles are very common in the ultrasounds of younger women, particularly in teenagers, as there is a natural abundance of follicles/eggs in this age group, which can in many cases exceed the threshold count for PCOS. In addition, during puberty, there is recruitment of many follicles as the ovary activates, without consistent ovulation as of yet, so girls in puberty naturally have a form of polycystic ovary. This, however, should resolve as girls begin to have regular ovulation and menstrual cycles.

So, for teenagers, it's always important to be cautious when looking at your ultrasound results. This is one important reason that we don't use the "cysts" alone to diagnose PCOS.

Conversely, women over thirty-five may have PCOS, but they have fewer follicles due to their egg bank becoming smaller with age and are less likely to have polycystic ovary appearance on ultrasound. As such, age really does matter when it comes to the "cystic" criteria. The good news is most women will decrease their likelihood of belonging to a "cystic" type as they get older.

Technology and Ovarian Cysts

Newer technology may be changing this long-held definition of what constitutes a "polycystic" ovary. In March 2013, a study concluded that a new threshold should be used to determine if a woman actually had cystic ovaries characteristic of PCOS.[2]

This is because diagnostic equipment has dramatically improved in its ability to detect follicles in the ovary. Over the past several years, many women *without* PCOS (and especially teenage girls who naturally have many follicles and are almost in a temporary PCOS-like state) were being diagnosed with polycystic ovaries on ultrasound, because the ultrasound technology has become so sensitive. Follicles that would have normally remained undetected by older equipment are now being picked up much more easily, increasing the number reported by the ultrasound technician.

The study concluded that a total of twenty-six follicles between two and nine millimeters long was a better marker of PCOS when using newer ultrasound technology. This study also noted that this threshold only applies to women between eighteen and thirty-five years of age. As previously mentioned, women under the age of eighteen naturally have larger amounts of follicles.

The Four Types Defined

From my point of view, the Rotterdam phenotypes are simply a compilation of some of the factors of PCOS that we need to know about in order to treat the disorder and really are not specific enough to form treatment guidelines over. For the purpose of treatment, I will be teaching you to identify your own unique factors, giving you the most customized treatment program possible. I believe that the Rotterdam phenotypes are important to know about to help you determine if you have PCOS in the first place and to understand more about the intensity of your PCOS.

As mentioned previously, women need to have two of the three Rotterdam criteria for a confirmed diagnosis. This leaves us with four unique types named, very aptly, the Rotterdam Phenotypes:

Type A and Type B are "classic PCOS" as defined by the NIH. Type C and Type D are "non-classic PCOS." Following are the new categories.

The Four PCOS Phenotypes

Type A: Delayed ovulation, hyperandrogenic, and polycystic ovaries on ultrasound

Type B: Delayed ovulation, hyperandrogenic, with normal ovaries on ultrasound

Type C: Hyperandrogenic, with polycystic ovaries on ultrasound, and with regular ovulation

Type D: Delayed ovulation, with polycystic ovaries on ultrasound, and without androgenic signs

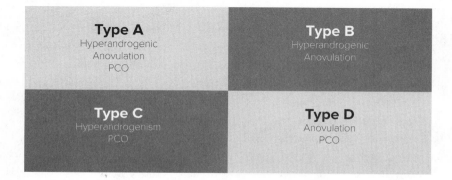

Figure 1-2: The Rotterdam Phenotypes of PCOS

A Diagnosis of Exclusion

PCOS is a diagnosis of exclusion. Therefore, other disorders that could cause these symptoms must be ruled out first. Other organizations strongly disagree with these types, especially Type D, the non-androgenic phenotype. An important international organization called the Androgen Excess and PCOS Society has concluded that, by definition, PCOS must include excess androgens. It's also possible, however, that Type D is simply a very mildly androgenic PCOS phenotype, as will be discussed in the next section.

The Stories of Molly and Lisa

Molly was a twenty-eight-year-old woman with PCOS who decided to improve her health after a particularly frustrating year dealing with the imbalances of her condition. She was approximately twenty pounds above the recommended weight suggested by her doctor, and her periods only arrived every three to four months. Molly had coarse hair on her chin and neck, and her ovaries looked like the classic "string of pearls" on ultrasound. Her diet was not the best; she lived a fast-paced life and ate out a lot. Nothing too terrible, but it was rare for her to cook her own meals. When Molly brought her concerns to her doctor, she was recommended a small dose of metformin, a diabetes drug commonly prescribed for PCOS. She followed this suggestion and changed her diet to completely remove processed foods and sugar. Over a period of four months, Molly successfully lost twenty pounds, and her periods began to cycle every twenty-nine days. Through treatment, she had moved from a Type A (most severe phenotype) to a Type C (a milder phenotype).

Lisa was a thirty-six-year-old woman with PCOS who also tended to get her periods every three to four months (an improvement from her younger years, when they were farther apart). Similarly to Molly, Lisa had some hair growth on her lip and chin (though it was mild in comparison), and her ultrasound revealed clusters of tiny follicles on each of her ovaries. After visiting her gynecologist, Lisa faithfully followed a diet and medication program similar to Molly's.

Her response was quite different, though: As had been the case for her whole life, Lisa found it exceptionally challenging to lose weight. After four months and a great deal of effort, she was only able to lose about five pounds.

Over the four-month time frame, Lisa's periods improved somewhat, but her cycle was still fifty-two days long. On ultrasound, however, her ovaries appeared to be healthier, now just below the cutoff for the cystic type. Through treatment, Lisa had moved from a Type A to a Type B.

What was the difference between these women's cases? Why did Molly improve so much when Lisa still struggled, despite following the same treatment?

Interestingly, Lisa was far more insulin resistant than Molly when blood tests were considered. Insulin resistance happens when the cells of the body don't respond normally in PCOS. It's one of the central factors in the condition, and the degree to which it is present can make a big difference in a woman's response to treatment. Chapter 3 describes insulin resistance in greater detail.

A more severe degree of insulin resistance was surely related to Lisa's difficulties in losing weight and was part of the reason she remained in one of the classic phenotypes. Insulin resistance is one of the first factors that we address in the 8 steps to healing your PCOS.

Frustrated with her lack of progress, Lisa visited her naturopathic doctor, who worked with her to change her insulin resistance factor. Although Lisa was already taking metformin, more help was needed since her insulin resistance markers were still elevated. She began to carefully follow a nutrition plan that managed her insulin resistance. (See chapter 9 and Appendix D for more information.)

At the same time, Lisa began an intensive exercise program and started taking supplements and herbs to improve her insulin resistance. After four months with this combined approach, Lisa began to cycle regularly every thirty days. She was elated: This was the first time in her life that she had achieved a regular cycle. Essentially, Lisa had moved from classic Type A PCOS to a full reversal of the syndrome. Over time, Lisa was able to wean herself off many of the supplements—even the metformin—and was able to maintain her healthy cycles with diet, exercise, and a few basic nutrients.

Every Woman Is Unique

This example goes to show that each woman is unique and may require different interventions to achieve a milder phenotype, or even better, to reverse PCOS entirely! As you can see, once only one criterion remains, or if your symptoms have cleared up, you can say that PCOS symptoms have been reversed in that the symptoms are no longer evident. That doesn't mean that you can take it easy now: Reversal is not the same as cured. You'll always have PCOS. It is a lifelong condition, and you will always have to take better care of yourself than those who don't have it. I like to look at that as a gift to your future self, knowing that the efforts you've made now will prevent many health problems for you in the future.

The take-home from this section really is this: The four phenotypes are certainly useful to understand. They are the diagnostic criteria for PCOS, and they determine how severe the condition is.

To effectively *treat* PCOS is a different matter. There are several important factors that need to be identified and addressed, and I hope to show you exactly how to achieve that in this book.

Now that we've talked about how each type is diagnosed, let's go through each of the four phenotypes and their differences according to current research.

Determining Your PCOS Type

To make it simple, you'll just need to determine which of the three criteria you have. If you don't know if you have one of the criteria for PCOS, that's OK. Take a deep breath. You'll still be able to use this book by following the 8 steps we go through in later chapters.

To determine your PCOS phenotype, ask yourself the following questions:

Hyperandrogenism

1. Do I have significant acne; hair growth on my chin, upper lip, stomach, upper thighs, upper arms, or back; or noticeable hair loss that is either diffuse or behind the front hairline that is not explained by another factor like an iron deficiency?

2. Or have I been tested for testosterone, DHEA, and androstenedione and are these numbers elevated? (See chapter 5 for a comprehensive discussion of the androgen hormones.)

Anovulation

1. Are my menstrual cycles irregular or usually thirty-five days long or longer?

2. Or do I experience difficulty in ovulation?

Polycystic Ovaries

1. Do I have multiple small follicles (more than twenty-six total) on my ovaries when I get an ultrasound?

To know if you belong to a cystic phenotype, you'll have to visit your doctor to have an ultrasound, so there may be women who don't know if they have ovarian "cysts." If you have one of the other two criteria and suspect that you may have PCOS, you should request an ultrasound. Remember that older women who may have had this factor in the past can outgrow this as their number of eggs decreases with maturity. Researchers now believe that when girls go through puberty (when the hormonal system temporarily enters a state that is very similar to PCOS), for most women, this passes. But for women with PCOS, it continues on. It's thought that PCOS may be similar to the hormonal situation of puberty not coming to its full completion. As such, using the cystic criteria to diagnose PCOS in a teenage girl is quite controversial, since many girls have ovaries with a PCOS type of appearance at this age.

You can now note which of the qualities you have and then combine them to determine your phenotype. If you are not able to get an ultrasound, but think you have PCOS, you can still use this book. You'll easily be able to determine your PCOS factors as we continue on, and that is where the real ability to work on your health comes from.

In the PCOS types that follow, you'll find that a variety of different hormones are mentioned. If you're unfamiliar with the hormone names and what they mean, you'll find a full discussion of the hormones and menstrual cycles in PCOS in chapter 6.

Phenotype A: "Classic" PCOS

This is the most severe phenotype of PCOS, containing all three of the criteria. Women with Type A "classic" PCOS have delayed ovulations and menstrual cycles, high androgens, and a "cystic" appearance to their ovaries.

Type A PCOS

- High androgens/androgenic signs
- Irregular periods/delayed ovulation
- Polycystic ovaries

This is also known as "classic" PCOS, and many women with this type tend to have a high body mass index and increased waist circumference. Elizabeth, from the opening of the chapter, is a Type A. Some patients who have Type A are of average weight or lean, and I believe that these patients may actually have the strongest genetic predisposition to PCOS overall, because the symptoms persist strongly, despite the metabolic benefits of lower weight. The good news is that when many women, even as they get older, change their diet and exercise or make changes to their hormonal health, they can move from Type A to another, milder phenotype.

Type As seem to have the most weight accumulated around their midsections and a high LH/FSH ratio on day three of their menstrual cycle.[3] They also tend to have the highest testosterone levels of all the types. This group may represent sixty percent of all PCOS patients.

Type As need to take very good care of their body as they age, as they definitely have a higher risk of developing metabolic diseases. There is more insulin resistance and a higher risk for both diabetes and heart disease.

Type As also have the highest anti-Mullerian hormone (AMH) levels of all the types. AMH is secreted by the follicles in the ovary and is used to measure the "number" of eggs left in the reserve. Most women with PCOS secrete higher than normal levels of AMH.

Type As often have the most menstrual irregularity as well. Many women in this category can go months without ovulation, and when periods do show up, they may not be actual periods and may instead be "breakthrough bleeds." Breakthrough bleeds happen when the endometrial lining builds up over a longer period of time, without the natural shedding of the menstrual cycle.

Type A women often have very low progesterone levels, as progesterone is only released after ovulation (which does not happen frequently). Without ovulation and progesterone, a woman will become estrogen dominant, and the lining of the uterus will thicken. After some time, the lining may begin to break down, causing spotting, irregular bleeding, and even bleeding that appears to be like a period, but which may be exceptionally painful, heavy, or clotted.

Type As have it rough! The good news is that most women can move out of type A and into another type by making changes to diet and lifestyle and by implementing natural medicine therapies.

Phenotype B: "Classic" PCOS

Type B, another "classic" form of PCOS, is similar to Type A PCOS, except that the ovaries do not contain cysts.

Type B PCOS

- High androgens
- Irregular periods/delayed ovulation
- Normal ovaries

Sophia, our tall woman with acne and irregular periods in the opening story, is a Type B. Women with Type B PCOS have irregular periods or delayed ovulation and signs of high androgens, such as hirsutism, acne, or hair loss. As is the case with Type A, they have the tendency to gain weight around their waistline and can have an increased body mass index. It's important to note that although there is an increased tendency toward weight gain in Type A and Type B, lean women can also be found in these types.

Studies have found that the main difference between Type A and Type B PCOS is that in Type B, AMH is lower, which makes sense because AMH correlates with the PCOS-like cysts of the ovary. As we mentioned earlier, with respect to cystic appearance reducing with age, Type B contains a greater number of older women.

Type B is not nearly as common as Type A and is found in only 8.4 percent of women with PCOS. According to Shroff, Types A and B share similar risks for diabetes and cardiovascular disease.[4]

Phenotype C: "Non-Classic" PCOS

Type C is one of the newer, "non-classic" forms of PCOS. Prior to Rotterdam, it may not have actually been considered a type of PCOS at all. In this type, we see elevated androgens and polycystic ovaries but regular menstrual cycles. This type of PCOS is also known as "ovulatory PCOS," and it represents one of the milder forms of PCOS.

Type C PCOS

- High androgens/androgenic signs
- Regular periods: thirty-five-day or shorter cycles/ovulation
- Polycystic ovaries

Many patients who have Type A classic PCOS will be able to move to Type C when they lose weight through dietary changes or work on insulin resistance. Women with Type C PCOS tend to have medium-level values of body mass index (BMI), waist circumference, and levels of androgens. Women with Type C often have lower LH/FSH ratios than Types A and B. Although Type Cs have higher androgen levels than women without PCOS, the androgens are not as high as in Type A.

Type Cs: You May Not Be Ovulating as Often as You Think!

One thing that is important to note is that women with Type C PCOS may actually not be ovulating within each cycle, although their period may arrive. A study found that many Type C women were only ovulating for a certain percentage of menstrual cycles.[5] What looked like a period was instead something called a breakthrough bleed—the result of incomplete ovulation.

For Type C, it is important to check Day 7 post-ovulation progesterone levels and/or to do basal body temperature (BBT) charting to determine how often true ovulations are occurring. Chapter 6 and Appendix A cover these topics in detail.

Marion's Story

Marion, a twenty-four-year-old Type C, tended to have her period every twenty-nine to thirty-four days, but occasionally her bleeding was exceptionally light. She was also experiencing significant hair loss just behind her hairline, as well as coarse hair growth on her chin. Marion was moderately slim and had been healthy her whole life, until she began to lose her hair. It was coming out at what seemed like a rapid pace, and Marion began to panic. Around the same time, she had an ultrasound from her gynecologist, who noted that her ovaries were filled with tiny follicles. She was then diagnosed with PCOS, and because her hair loss and hirsutism fit the androgenic pattern, she fit into Type C. I worked with Marion to help reduce her androgen levels and regulate her hormones. Marion made the commitment to give up her addiction to sugar and sweet treats. Although Marion's cycles were never exceptionally delayed, with treatment, they became regular at thirty-day intervals. Over time, Marion's hair grew back beautifully as well.

Phenotype D PCOS: "Non-Classic" PCOS

Type D PCOS

- Normal androgens
- Irregular periods/delayed ovulation
- Polycystic ovaries

Now here is where it gets interesting: Type D is the most controversial type of PCOS. Until Rotterdam, women with this type were not considered to have PCOS at all, and even now, many experts have argued that Type D is not a true PCOS. It's quite possible that this category may eventually disappear altogether, but I would like to cover it, as I believe that there are a small number of women in this category who may be undiagnosed.

Women with this type of PCOS have no androgenic signs and normal androgen levels. They do, however, have polycystic ovaries and irregular periods or delayed ovulation. Along with Type C, Type D has more tendency toward being of lower body mass index and less insulin resistance.[6] Many lean women with mild PCOS not previously detected fit into this category, particularly after stopping the birth control pill. That being said, it's important to remember that lean women with PCOS can fit into any phenotype.

Type D: Removing Other Possibilities

In order to be diagnosed with Type D (or any type of PCOS for that matter), the other disorders that mimic PCOS must be ruled out first. This can be achieved with proper bloodwork and testing. Again, if one of these other conditions is found to be the cause of your symptoms, you may not have PCOS.

Disorders That Mimic PCOS

- Hypothyroidism

- High prolactin levels

- Hypothalamic amenorrhea (a disconnect in the brain-pituitary-ovary axis)

- Non-classical congenital adrenal hyperplasia (a rare genetic condition of the adrenals)

A Middle Ground

Although there has been much argument about Type D, there may actually be a middle ground between the two positions. According to Guastella, Longo, and Carmina, Type Ds in fact *do* have a very mild androgen excess *when compared to women without PCOS*. In Type D, androgens are within the normal range but still may be slightly higher than in women without PCOS.

It's also been found that when women with Type D are stimulated with certain medications, they will in fact produce excess androgens compared to women who don't have PCOS. Given that measuring androgens in the blood can be very challenging (more about this in chapter 5), this type may simply be the mildest variant of PCOS.

Mina's Story

Mina was a twenty-four-year-old woman who only had periods every four months. She went to a gynecologist who performed an ultrasound for her, and it was determined that she had polycystic-appearing ovaries. When the doctor ran bloodwork, her testosterone and androgen levels were completely normal. Mina had no acne or male-pattern hair growth: She's a Type D.

In Mina's case, because she has many follicles in her ovary, we consider her to be *potentially* hyperandrogenic. Although this is one of the milder variants of PCOS, Mina would respond best to the specific treatments aimed at improving ovarian health and at enhancing ovulations.

As a general rule, women with Type D are not as insulin resistant as other phenotypes. They are more likely to have a normal BMI and normal waist circumference and often fall into the "lean" PCOS group (though it's important to remember that lean women can be in any category).

When it comes to hormones, Type Ds have an increased LH to FSH ratio and an increased LH. This is may be why ovulation doesn't happen regularly in this type. In many cases, women in Types A or B can move to Type D as their PCOS improves.

It's important to note that studies have shown that women in all PCOS phenotypes, even Type Ds, display at least mild insulin resistance when challenged with glucose or carbohydrates. In each case, however, the degree of insulin resistance is quite different, and the treatment should be tailored to each woman's needs, which we will go into great detail about very soon.

What Influences Your PCOS Phenotype

We are all unique. This is why the treatment that works for Sophia may not work for Elizabeth. Each woman with PCOS has a unique set of imbalances, or as I call them, "factors" that need to be addressed. This where there may be some stumbling blocks in the current treatment of the disorder where a one-size–fits-all approach is often used. In this book, I hope to provide some tools that I have developed through my clinical experience in treating women step-by-step by their unique factors.

The following sections address the elements that can influence the PCOS phenotype that a woman has.

Factors That Influence Your PCOS Type

- Age
- Weight
- Environment
- Genetics
- Socio-Emotions

Age

Young women naturally have more follicles in their ovaries and are more likely to be in a "cystic" phenotype. This is particularly the case for teenagers. As women age, the number of follicles in the ovary naturally decline. The newer threshold for twenty-six follicles does not apply to women under eighteen and over thirty-five for this very reason.

Fortunately, another main PCOS problem gets better with age: the levels of the androgenic hormones, such as testosterone and DHEA. As such, a woman may move from one of the more severe phenotypes, such as A, to one of the less severe phenotypes, such as C, as she gets older. *So yes, the hormonal and reproductive problems of PCOS can actually improve as a woman gets older! That's* great, right?

It is, but there is some bad news, too: It's important to know that the metabolic risks of PCOS, like cardiovascular disease and type 2 diabetes, actually *increase* with age (see Appendix C).

Weight

Weight is one of the most important central factors that can determine the severity of PCOS. Weight gain (not including that of lean muscle) promotes insulin resistance, and insulin resistance is associated with more classic types, such as Type A or Type B. Weight loss, particularly loss of inches at the waist, can often easily move a woman to a milder phenotype. The opposite is also true: Gaining weight, especially around the waist, can move a woman from a "non-classic" type, such as C, to a "classic" type, such as A or B.

Studies show that women should aim for an abdominal circumference of thirty-five inches or less to achieve a milder phenotype. In those with smaller frames, such as Southeast Asian women, the recommended abdominal circumference to reduce insulin resistance is thirty-two inches or less.

Epigenetics and Environment

Epigenetics are when the expression of your DNA changes in response to something in the environment. Yes, that's right—your genetics are changeable! A few epigenetic associations have been made with PCOS: Most notably, animal studies have found that babies exposed to a high androgen environment (such as in Mom's bloodstream) during pregnancy seem to be more prone to PCOS as adults. This may be in part why PCOS can be passed on in families.

With respect to the environment, if a woman is exposed to toxic xenoestrogenic products, such as plastics, PCBs, and other toxins (included in the environmental section in chapter 8), this may exacerbate PCOS hormonal imbalances and even induce PCOS in the next generation.

Genetics

Some women are just more prone to more severe phenotypes of the condition than others, despite the changes they may make in their diet because of their lifestyle and hormonal factors. More and more evidence is being produced confirming that PCOS is a genetic disorder.

Socio-Emotional Factors

This may sound like an unusual category, but socio-emotional factors can actually contribute to the type of PCOS a woman has. It is unlikely that this alone can move her from one category to another, but there is good indication to suggest that stress and emotional health play a role in the severity of PCOS. Stress and mood are discussed in great detail in chapter 4. Women with PCOS often have higher-than-average cortisol levels, which can trigger a variety of hormonal imbalances.

Social factors, such as cultural and familial diet styles and the social influence of exercise, may influence the phenotype of a woman with PCOS through the types of activities that she does and the types of food that she eats. For example, in some cultures, including Southeast Asia and Latin America, carbohydrates are a mainstay of the diet, which leads to an increased predisposition to more classic forms of PCOS.

Final Notes about the PCOS Types

What I'm about to say may surprise you: It's really important to know that the particular "type" is not what matters most. When it comes down to it, we all want to be healthier, happier, more fertile, and have great hormone balance and good skin, right?

From my experience, I've found that working through my system, step by step, using your unique PCOS factors, will help move you from a more severe type to a milder one, or even to a full reversal of your PCOS symptoms and reduction of risks. So, if you haven't had an ultrasound of your ovaries and are not sure what type you really are, that's OK. Keep reading: The best information to heal your PCOS is in the upcoming chapters.

Your PCOS factors may be very different than they were ten years ago, and five years from now, they will likely be different again. My goal is to look at PCOS not as a static disease but rather as a dynamic disorder that affects women's bodies in unique ways as they pass through life.

My dream is for all women with PCOS to be treated as individuals and to have each woman's case looked at with the detail that they deserve. A careful look at your unique characteristics gives you the power to begin the process of reversing your PCOS. So let us begin by looking at the first step.

Chapter 2

STEP 1. ADDRESS INFLAMMATION

Happiness is not a matter of intensity but of balance, order, rhythm and harmony.

—THOMAS MERTON

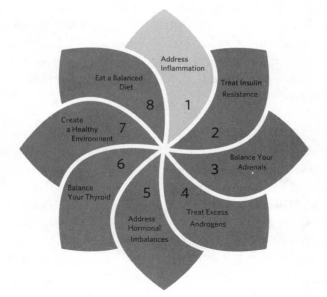

Aisha had just turned thirty-three years old. She'd been struggling with PCOS her whole life but had only just been diagnosed, prior to going through difficulties conceiving her baby. She had never had regular cycles and suffered from relentless hirsutism. Despite following the same diet and exercise programs as her friends, she never saw the results they were able to achieve. She had tried birth control pills in an attempt to regulate her period, only to find that they caused her excruciating migraines. In addition to all of the challenges she faced with PCOS, she developed an autoimmune condition known as Hashimoto's thyroiditis after giving birth to her first baby, which left her feeling unable to function and exhausted. Aisha was tired and moody. She suffered from insomnia and headaches, and her periods just never seemed to be predictable. How could all of this happen to her?

Inflammation: What Is It Exactly?

Inflammation is a hallmark factor of PCOS. Evidence has mounted showing that chronic low-grade inflammation is not just a side effect of PCOS, as thought previously. It is the central factor in the condition. Inflammation has a purpose within our bodies. It's the secretion of special chemicals by the cells of our immune system that can activate different healing processes, attract other immune cells to help out, and destroy foreign invaders like viruses or bacteria. It's basically our body's chemical way of protecting itself. We want inflammation under certain circumstances—like if we have a wound or an infection. However, what we don't want is to have inflammation all of the time.

Inflammatory chemicals are made to damage cells of invaders, but they can also damage our own cells if left unchecked. Having chronic inflammation in our bodies can disrupt our hormones and cause premature aging. Chronic inflammation can also damage our egg quality and intestinal health and can even cause depression and anxiety. As women with PCOS, we need to address this key issue in order to fully heal.

Cytokines

The entire inflammatory process is modulated by special chemical signals that are secreted by immune cells. These are known as cytokines. Some of the common cytokines are TNF-alpha, IL-6, IL-18, IFN-g, and IL-10. Cytokines are helpful in most instances. For example, if there is a viral invader, the immune cells release cytokines, signaling to the rest of the immune system that there is a battle to fight.

However, in PCOS, these cytokines are secreted constantly at a low level. This creates a variety of unwanted symptoms, as inflammation can directly act on the ovary to cause the production of testosterone[1] and on the fat cells to cause insulin resistance.[2] This phenomenon is known as chronic low-grade inflammation, and it is a pervasive and central factor of PCOS.

Lipotoxicity

PCOS has recently been linked to different abnormalities in the way that our fat cells behave and how fatty acids are metabolized in our bodies. To a certain point, our fat cells are great at storing the excess energy we consume. When there is an excess of energy input within our fat cells, the cells will spill free fatty acids out into our circulation.

Other cells in our circulation don't have the capacity to store fatty acids, so the excess remains in the bloodstream. This is very dangerous, as these fatty acids can cause tissue damage. This damage can occur in the liver, kidneys, heart, pancreas, and in many other organs in the body.

Another issue is that adipose (fatty) tissue has poor circulation. As such, the fat cells (adipocytes) often die off, especially in the inner areas of fatty tissue. The more fatty tissue that is present, the more this happens. This is known as fat necrosis. As the cells die off, the immune system comes in to clear things out. But in doing so, it is constantly releasing cytokines to do its job. This causes a chronic state of low-grade inflammation originating in the fatty tissue, known as lipotoxicity (see Figure 2-1).[3]

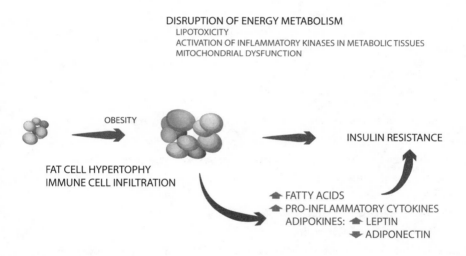

Figure 2-1: Lipotoxicity

Whether lean or heavy, women with PCOS have higher levels of a certain type of lipotoxic fatty acid, called non-esterified fatty acids (NEFA). When lipotoxicity happens in the tissues of the body that are insulin sensitive, it can contribute to insulin resistance.

In fact, it's now thought that lipotoxicity may be a central cause of insulin resistance in our tissues. It's been known for a long time that people who have inflammatory conditions, like rheumatoid arthritis, are more prone to type 2 diabetes, as inflammation promotes insulin resistance. As such, it really must be addressed first and foremost in any plan to reverse PCOS symptoms.

A study by Frank González in 2012 found that lipotoxicity and NEFAs cause androgens to be released from the ovaries of women with PCOS. Part of the issue with the damaging effects of lipotoxity is that there are limited ways to dispose of these fatty acids. Many of the detoxification pathways depend on antioxidants to quench the damaging free radicals that are generated as our bodies try to dispose of the fatty acids. If our disposal pathways are strong, we can deal with more of these fatty acids and reduce their damaging effects on our insulin pathways.

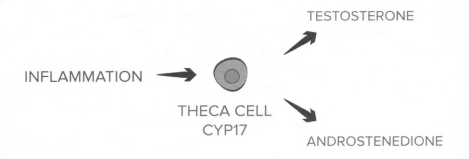

Figure 2-2: Inflammation-Androgen

The Difference between Inflammation and Autoimmunity

Autoimmune diseases are more common in women with PCOS. Autoimmunity occurs when our immune cells produce antibodies against our own tissues. It's normal for our immune cells to do this, as this is our immune system's way of being able to adapt to new influences. However, there are also cells in the immune system that should keep the antibodies to our own tissues in check.

In autoimmune disease, these processes go unchecked, and our immune systems mount an attack against our own tissue in a similar manner to how they would attack a bacteria or a virus. When an autoimmune disease is active, there is a lot of inflammation. The immune cells that are activated by autoimmune processes produce many of the same chemicals (cytokines) that we see in the general inflammatory state of PCOS. The names of some of these chemicals are NF-kappa B, TNF-alpha, and IL-6. In true autoimmune disease, there is often an additional chemical that comes into play called IL-17.

These chemicals are very harmful to our body when they are left unchecked. Typically, our immune system should reside in a state where it is sensitive and responds to the environment—activating to defend against infections and turning off overactive responses when needed. In PCOS, this entire pattern is disrupted, and we have what is referred to as a state of chronic low-grade inflammation. So, what should we do about this?

Tests for Inflammation

There are some tests you can take to determine the level of inflammation in your body. These include high-sensitivity C-reactive protein (hs-CRP) and erythrocyte sedimentation rate (ESR), which are two nonspecific markers of inflammation in the body that tell you that inflammation is there but not what is causing it.

Hs-CRP

This protein is a general marker of inflammation. Often used to assess for risk of cardiovascular disease, it's a test I have often found elevated in women with PCOS. The higher the hs-CRP level is, the more intense the inflammation. Please note that if you have a cold or the flu or any other cause for inflammation at the time of the test, it could be falsely elevated, so testing at a time when you are at your baseline is highly recommended.

ESR

This is a relatively simple test used to detect general inflammation. It is particularly good at picking up inflammation associated with autoimmune diseases. However, it can also be high during other inflammatory states like infection, so it should only be tested in a baseline state. While ESR and hs-CRP do not reveal the cause of inflammation, these inexpensive tests can pick up and track the progress of an inflammatory condition.

Tests for True Autoimmunity

There are a multitude of tests for true autoimmune diseases, and it is outside of the scope of this book to cover all of them. I will, however, include the most common antibodies that may be positive in women who have autoimmune diseases. These include the anti-thyroid antibodies, antinuclear antibodies, and the celiac antibodies.

Anti-Tg, Anti-TPO

The two most common antibodies that attack the thyroid gland are anti-thyroglobulin (anti-Tg) and anti-thyroid peroxidase (anti-TPO). As Hashimoto's thyroiditis is the most common cause of hypothyroidism and is the number one autoimmune disease overall, this test is one of the more likely markers to come up positive when screening for autoimmunity. As women with PCOS have an increased incidence of Hashimoto's, it's definitely a good idea to have these markers screened.

ANA

Antinuclear antibody (ANA) is one of the primary tests used to identify autoimmune diseases. It may be positive in a variety of autoimmune disorders, including conditions like lupus and Sjogren's syndrome. However, it may also be high without a detectable autoimmune disease, which can be a sign that an autoimmune disease could develop in the future.

Celiac Disease

Blood tests can be done to rule out celiac disease, although the gold standard is the small intestinal biopsy to look for the telltale signs of destruction of the tiny microvilli that line the intestinal wall. You must be consuming gluten to get accurate results for celiac disease through either blood or intestinal biopsy. The blood tests for celiac disease include the following: Tissue transglutaminase IgA (the most commonly tested), endomysial antibodies, and deaminated gliadin peptide antibodies.

Some advanced labs offer functional immune testing, which can pick up the markers commonly found in inflammatory states, including TNF-alpha, IFN-g, IL-6, and IL-17.

How to Treat Inflammation

When your test results show you have inflammation, you can either try conventional methods or natural ones. We will cover both methods in this section to give you the broadest understanding of the options available to you.

Conventional Methods

In conventional medicine, inflammation is often addressed in women with PCOS through the use of metformin or other insulin-sensitizing agents, since insulin resistance promotes inflammation and vice versa. For more information on metformin, please see the chapter on insulin resistance.

Steroids

In patients who have autoimmune diseases, immune-suppressing steroid medications can be prescribed. These have a variety of negative side effects, are harmful to the liver, cause weight gain, and are generally only used in more serious autoimmune disorders.

Newer Immune Medications

Low-dose naltrexone (LDN) is a newer and gentler option used in the treatment of autoimmune diseases. At higher doses, naltrexone is a treatment that blocks the opioid receptors and was originally used to help people overcome addictions. However, recent research has found that the effects of naltrexone are different at small doses, around one-tenth of the original doses used. At smaller doses, naltrexone has anti-inflammatory effects and also appears to help the body produce more of its own beta endorphins. Women with PCOS often have dysfunction of the hormonal system that can be improved through maintaining good levels of beta endorphins, which we discuss more in chapter 6. In addition to this, LDN seems to calm down immune cells called microglia. These cells, when chronically active, may cause chronic inflammation in the body. LDN has been associated with lowering levels of the inflammatory chemicals TNF-alpha and IL-6 and overall markers of inflammation, such as ESR.

Research also suggests that naltrexone can assist women with PCOS, presumably because of its benefits in reducing inflammation, which is central to the condition. One study investigated women with PCOS who were resistant to clomiphene and found that LDN was able to restore sensitivity to clomiphene and induce ovulation in the majority of the women studied. It also found that the women on LDN had reductions in insulin, improvements in FSH/LH ratios, and reduced levels of testosterone.

That being said, most women with PCOS can address inflammation completely with diet, lifestyle, and natural supplements, so let's explore that now!

Natural Ways to Manage PCOS Inflammation

As PCOS has inflammation at its center, all women with this condition have increased baseline cytokines. That being said, there are many other processes in the body that can add to this inflammation. When looking at natural approaches to inflammation, we want to address all of the potential areas where inflammation may arise. This may include addressing autoimmune diseases, managing food reactions, or healing insulin resistance.

Insulin Counting and an Anti-Inflammatory Diet

The first step in dealing with inflammation in PCOS is to address the particular hormones, namely insulin, that trigger even more inflammation, perpetuating a vicious cycle. As such, the insulin counting recommendations in chapter 3 are very helpful in mitigating inflammation, particularly in women who tend to carry extra weight around their abdomen.

In addition, the recommended foods in chapter 9 are primarily anti-inflammatory in nature. Following these recommendations will benefit all women with PCOS, whether lean or not. This anti-inflammatory approach removes dairy and sugar and focuses on whole, real, natural food whenever possible.

Leaky Gut and Inflammation

It's here that I want to talk about the health of our digestive system. It's important to know that a major part of immune system development occurs right underneath the cells of the small intestine, in tissue known as the GALT, or gut-associated lymphoid tissue. The GALT is where new immune cells grow and develop to be released into the bloodstream. The intestinal cells should provide a sealed barrier, protecting the bloodstream from the contents of the intestine. Within the intestine, there are nutrients, partially digested foods, bacteria, and a variety of different chemicals that we may have ingested. None of this should have direct access to the immune system.

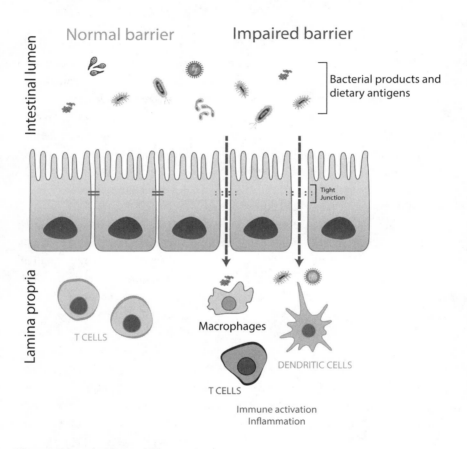

Figure 2-3: Intestinal Permeability

However, if the barrier of the intestine becomes broken, many of the contents of the intestine will leak through, coming into contact with the immune cells underneath. When the intestinal barrier is no longer intact, this is known as "leaky gut," or by the more scientific term increased intestinal permeability. The immune cells will do their job by activating in response to these foreign particles, creating inflammation. The inflammation created by the immune cells not only disrupts the health of the body, but can also disrupt the development of the other immune cells, creating an increase in autoimmune disease and dysfunctional immune responses.

As such, keeping this intestinal barrier intact is very important when it comes to keeping inflammation at bay. Inflammatory responses from leaky gut add on to what is already present in PCOS.

Symptoms of Leaky Gut

The signs and symptoms of leaky gut include bloating, indigestion, food sensitivities, inflammatory bowel disease, autoimmune disease, thyroid disease, malabsorption of nutrients, inflamed skin, depression, and anxiety. In fact, many people who have chronic inflammation also have leaky gut.

How You Can Minimize Leaky Gut

One very basic and simple thing that you can do to heal leaky gut is to eliminate or reduce gluten in your diet. When intestinal cells are exposed to gliadin (a major component of gluten), they release a substance known as zonulin.[4] Zonulin is the compound responsible for opening the barriers between the intestinal cells. In people who have celiac disease, an autoimmune reaction to wheat, the release of zonulin is intense, and the intestinal barrier becomes so damaged that it takes a very long time to repair. In those without celiac disease, depending on the level of sensitivity to gluten, the repair happens more quickly. Recent research has found that there are many individuals who have gluten sensitivity and increased zonulin levels but who don't have celiac disease, so always listen to your body and consider how you feel after eating gluten.[5]

Other aggravating factors that contribute to leaky gut are food allergies. The most common food allergies include dairy, wheat, corn, and soy. However, it's possible to be allergic to anything, and when you have leaky gut, as more foods access the immune system in an undigested form, more food allergies can develop.

Generally, I recommend an anti-inflammatory diet, which you can read more about in chapter 9. However, if you have significant reactions to food or are not able to get to the bottom of what foods may be aggravating you, food allergy testing or elimination diets may be helpful.

Food Allergy Testing

Most types of food allergy testing measure IgG antibodies, a specific type of antibody that is elevated in patients who have leaky gut. This type of allergy testing has come under criticism as the results may not always correlate with actual food reactions, but instead may be related in some cases to immune system exposure to the foods currently being eaten. As such, people with leaky gut syndrome may come back with many IgG food reactions on testing. As IgG also signifies that the immune system has come into contact with a food, it doesn't necessarily correlate to a food reaction. However, many people do find it helpful and have had good results from eliminating reactive foods from this testing procedure. There are also newer and more promising food reactivity tests for those with significant allergies or autoimmunity. These involve testing for immune reactivity with both IgA and IgG, along with reactivity to various breakdown particles within food, heat modified protein reactivity, and combined food reactions.

Elimination Diet

This is, in my opinion, a very good way to assess food intolerance and is particularly helpful for those who have a true autoimmune condition in combination with PCOS. It is challenging, but it is an affordable method of determining your reactions to different foods. Keep in mind that food reactions can change over time. A food that once aggravated you may not bother you in the future. One of my favorite plans that can help identify major food intolerances is the autoimmune paleo (AIP) protocol.

AIP involves an elimination phase consisting of the most common aggravating foods, including grains, dairy, sugar, nuts, seeds, alcohol, and the nightshade vegetables like potatoes, tomatoes, and eggplant. After a period of elimination (often at least four weeks), the foods are reintroduced carefully, one at a time, and reactions are noted. If there is no reaction to a particular food, it can be added back into the diet. I've included some wonderful websites on AIP in Appendix E. There are a variety of other gut-friendly diets, including the specific carbohydrate diet (SCD) and the gut and psychology syndrome (GAPS) diet, which are popular for those with significant intestinal issues.

PCOS-Friendly Supplements to Minimize Inflammation

Now that we've worked with the underlying hormonal and nutritional causes of inflammation in PCOS (i.e., metabolism and the gut), I'd like to introduce some of my favorite supplements that help with the general inflammation we often see in the condition.

Resveratrol

Resveratrol is one of my favorite anti-inflammatory supplements for women with PCOS. It has been found to minimize the secretion of the cytokines TNF-alpha and IL-6 and can also reduce NF-kappa B, which is one of the main inflammatory pathway signalers in the body.[6] When looking for resveratrol, trans-resveratrol is the form that has been associated with health benefits. Typical dosages of trans-resveratrol range from 100 to 250 mg per day.

Omega-3 Fatty Acids

Found in fish oils and flaxseed oil, omega-3 fatty acids have many benefits for women with PCOS. Omega-3 fatty acids and, in particular, eicosapentaenoic acid (EPA) are anti-inflammatory in action, reducing most of the inflammatory markers, such as TNF-alpha, IL-6 and IL-17.[7] It's important to note that I recommend fish oil over flaxseed oil, as it is the EPA in fish oil that has a strong anti-inflammatory action. Flaxseed oil contains alpha-linolenic acid (ALA), an omega-3 fatty acid that the body must convert to EPA, which only happens in very small amounts.

I usually recommend in the range of 1,000 mg of EPA per day. This is different than 1,000 mg total omega-3 fatty acid, so be sure to read labels carefully! The anti-inflammatory effects of omega-3 fatty acids are dose-dependent. Omega-3 fatty acids also increase the beneficial adiponectin protein. Read through the chapter on nutrition to learn more about how to choose a good quality omega-3 fatty acid.

Bioflavonoids—Grape Seed Extract, Pine Bark Extract, Green Tea EGCG

Then we enter the world of the bioflavonoids. These are actually some of the earth's best natural weapons against harmful inflammatory chemicals. They all reduce NF-kappa B, calming overactive immune responses.[8] They can decrease TH1 cytokines like TNF-alpha.[9] The catechin EGCG and grape seed extract are very helpful in increasing the regulatory T cells, or Tregs, that many patients who have autoimmune disease are deficient in.[10] Tregs help to calm and control overactive immune responses. To increase your dietary intake of these natural weapons against inflammation, I recommend eating foods rich in bioflavonoids, such as dark-colored berries, and drinking green tea. For women who have significant inflammation, there are also potent supplement extracts available for a more powerful effect. Bioflavonoids have also been found to increase levels of the beneficial compound adiponectin that is secreted from our fat cells.

Typical doses of grape seed extract, EGCG, or pycnogenol range from 50 to 200 mg per day.

Systemic Enzymes

Systemic enzymes are another safe and effective anti-inflammatory supplement. These are often extracted from fruits, such as pineapple and papaya (bromelain and papain), and in some instances from silkworms (serrapeptase). These enzymes are best taken on an empty stomach. If taken with a meal, they will exert their enzymatic effects on breaking down your food rather than entering your bloodstream, minimizing inflammation there. They have the ability to reduce IFN gamma and increase the regulatory cytokines that keep autoimmunity at bay.[11] Systemic enzymes do have a slight ability to thin the blood, so they should never be combined with other blood thinners without a doctor's supervision. That being said, for women with PCOS who are more at risk for blood clots, this may be a helpful benefit.

Dosing for systemic enzymes varies depending on the combination, but they must be taken on an empty stomach for full effects.

Glutathione and N-Acetyl Cysteine
Glutathione is the master antioxidant within our cells. It patrols the cell and quenches free radicals that can do damage within. As you can imagine, for women who have a lot of inflammation, having sufficient glutathione can be exceptionally protective to their cells.

Knowing that inflammation triggers the cellular damage that causes insulin resistance, this is perhaps why anti-inflammatory nutrients such as N-acetyl cysteine (NAC) protect against insulin resistance and benefit women with PCOS.[12]

N-acetyl cysteine is a proven precursor to glutathione: When you take it as an oral supplement, cellular levels of glutathione increase. Several studies suggest that NAC is a beneficial supplement for PCOS, improving ovulation, reducing androgens, and mitigating insulin resistance all through this antioxidant function. The typical dose for N-acetyl cysteine for PCOS is 600 mg three times per day.

Other forms of glutathione have not been absorbed well orally until recent years, when new forms were created. These include N-acetyl glutathione and liposomal glutathione, which have both in preliminary research been found to enter the cell and increase glutathione levels.

Curcumin
Curcumin is a powerful anti-inflammatory supplement extracted from the popular golden spice turmeric. One caveat is that it probably shouldn't be used in women who are trying to conceive, as it has also been investigated as a contraceptive.[13] Outside of that, however, it's been well proven to have numerous potent anti-inflammatory actions.[14, 15]

Typical doses of curcumin range from 50 to 500 mg per day. When it comes to choosing a curcumin supplement, turmeric powder won't give you enough. Not only is curcumin in its raw form poorly absorbed, but turmeric also contains only three percent curcumin, which doesn't even come close to matching the amounts used in research. If you want to derive benefits from curcumin, you must use one of the following absorbable forms: curcumin paired with piperine (black pepper), nanoparticle theracurmin, curcumin phytosomes with phosphatidylcholine, or water-soluble curcumin. Looking for these types of extracts can ensure this herb makes it into your system, where it can do its work!

Vitamin D

Vitamin D is essential for women with PCOS. I've called it one of the most important nutrients for women with PCOS for good reason. Therapeutic doses of vitamin D can be anti-inflammatory in nature. Studies have found that vitamin D can decrease TNF-alpha and IL-6, which is definitely beneficial for PCOS-mediated inflammation. It's interesting to note that many autoimmune diseases are associated with vitamin D deficiency. This may be because vitamin D is crucial for the formation of T regulatory cells. These cells are the calmers of the immune system, keeping it in check when it becomes overactive. I typically recommend having vitamin D serum levels checked and then supplementing these levels according to specific needs. For women who have no access to testing, a dosing of approximately 3,000 IU is safe to take daily.

Healing the Gut

For those who have a true autoimmune disease or digestive symptoms like bloating, indigestion, or reflux, there are nutrients that can be used to heal the gut, minimizing the overall inflammatory load on the body. These include probiotics, digestive enzymes, L-glutamine, N-acetyl glucosamine, and zinc.

Probiotics

One of the most researched topics in gut health, probiotics have powerful evidence with respect to their benefits in humans. Depending on the case, different probiotics can be recommended. Often you'll want to choose a quality strain, including at least both a lactobacillus strain and a bifidus strain. Multi-strain probiotics can also be quite beneficial. For those with autoimmune diseases, there are probiotics with proven anti-inflammatory action, including specific strains of *L. rhamnosus*, *B. infantis*, and *L. plantarum*.[16] The gut microbiome also has an important effect on metabolism, which will be discussed in the chapter on insulin resistance.

Digestive Enzymes

If you are suffering from bloating or gas after eating, you may have trouble digesting the foods you are eating. Part of the digestive process requires sufficient enzymes, which are produced by the pancreas to break down food. A broad-spectrum digestive enzyme, either plant based or with actual pancreatin (from pancreatic extract), can be used to assist the breakdown of foods in the digestive tract.

L- Glutamine

L-glutamine is a common amino acid that is the preferred fuel of the intestinal cells. In leaky gut, the intestinal cells can use L-glutamine to repair and regenerate, improving recovery time. It also protects the cells of the intestine from damage, reducing leaky gut and acting as a barrier to bacteria and other irritants. Typical doses of L-glutamine range from 5 to10 grams per day.

N-Acetyl Glucosamine

This powerful nutrient can calm irritation in the digestive tract. It also helps the cells of the intestine to produce its glycoprotein cover, which protects them from irritants. Typical doses range from 500 mg to 6 grams per day, depending on the level of intestinal inflammation.

Zinc

An important nutrient for intestinal health, zinc can actually tighten and strengthen the junctions between the cells.[17] Directly helpful for minimizing the leakiness of the gut, it can speed the rate at which the cells are replaced, and its anti-inflammatory actions are protective against allergies or irritants. Doses for zinc range from 5 to 30 mg per day, and higher doses of zinc should always be complexed with copper (usually 15 mg zinc to 2 mg copper) to protect against copper deficiency.

Chapter 3

STEP 2. TREAT INSULIN RESISTANCE

The strongest oak tree of the forest is not the one that is pro-
tected from the storm and hidden from the sun. It's the one that
stands in the open where it is compelled to struggle for its exis-
tence against the winds and rains and the scorching sun.

—NAPOLEON HILL

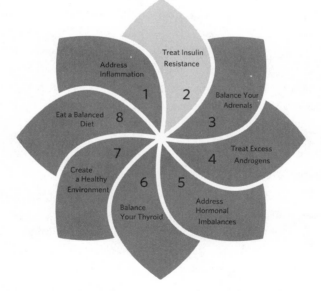

Alice had always struggled with her weight. Since she was a young child, she carried a little extra around the middle compared to her friends. As she continued through her preteen and teen years, she gradually gained more weight. She seemed to gain mostly around her abdomen, while her friends gained weight around their hips and thighs.

Alice also struggled with intense cravings for carbohydrates. In particular, she craved breads, pasta, and sweets and chocolates. Between meals, she would become shaky and would need to snack to get through her day. In time, she also noticed dark, velvety pigmentation in the folds of skin behind her neck and skin tags. When she turned thirty, Alice began feeling dizzy and strange after eating. What was wrong? Alice felt that she could definitely stand to lose a few pounds, but the diets that she attempted over the years always ended in her losing weight initially and then gaining all of it back plus more afterward.

She had been diagnosed with PCOS at age twenty-five and had been told repeatedly that she should lose weight to improve her menstrual cycles. This was frustrating: She simply could not lose weight like the other people she knew. There had to be a reason.

Alice, like many other women diagnosed with PCOS, suffers from insulin resistance—one of the most important factors that can intensely affect PCOS and one of the factors that carries forward throughout a woman's entire life.

· · · · ·

Insulin is an important hormone that helps us store energy. It helps our bodies move nutrients (like carbohydrates or proteins) from the bloodstream into the cells of our bodies. Insulin moves nutrients in only one direction—into the cells—for storage or immediate use.

When we eat carbohydrates like starches, they are broken down into simple sugars and are then taken up into our bloodstream. Our blood sugar rises at this point. High blood sugar is not good for our health, so our bodies have a special mechanism for controlling it, and that mechanism is insulin. The pancreas notices our increased blood sugar and responds by secreting insulin, which takes the sugar and moves it into our cells.

Insulin Sensitivity

You may have noticed that blood sugar regulation depends on the cells of our body being sensitive to insulin. This means that the cells can recognize and respond to insulin by pulling in the extra sugar from the bloodstream, storing it, and keeping blood sugar at the optimal level. Our cells need to be able to listen to insulin's message to keep our blood sugar regulated tightly.

As we all know, high blood sugar is related to a variety of chronic diseases. For example, it can damage our liver, pancreas, brain, heart, and eyes. High blood sugar also causes inflammation.

Before we learn more about insulin resistance, you'll need to learn about the main players in your metabolism: the who's who of the world of energy regulation that goes on in our bodies every moment of every day.

Glycogen

Once our cells have taken glucose out of the bloodstream with the help of insulin, it can be stored as energy that can be used later when needed. The primary place to store glucose is in the liver and muscles, as a compound known as glycogen. In the liver, glycogen can be readily converted back into glucose any time extra energy is needed.

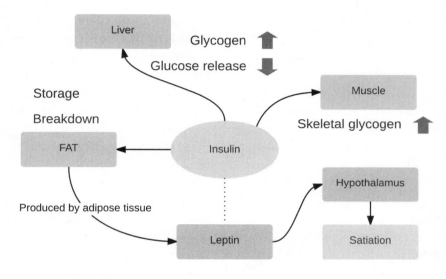

Figure 3-1: Insulin resistance causes leptin resistance.

Glycogen that is stored in the liver is often used when you exercise and when you fast (like when you sleep). In fact, glycogen acts almost like a "tank" of fuel that can be pulled upon when needed.

Once the liver is full of glycogen, if more carbohydrates are consumed, there is no place to store them. At this point, the body will need to go through another pathway to store the excess energy. Your liver takes that extra glucose and turns it into a special type of fat called triglyceride.

High triglycerides are not good. They are associated with increased body fat storage and increased free fatty acids (think: inflammation) floating around in our bloodstream. They are not good for our cardiovascular health or overall health. Women with PCOS often have high triglycerides. This is related to insulin resistance and excessive storage of carbohydrates.

Leptin

In the past, it was thought that adipose (fat) tissue was largely inert and was simply a storage tissue to hold excess energy the body didn't need at the time. We now know that adipose tissue is an active organ, and it secretes different signals in response to the environment. Leptin is one of the signals secreted by our fat calls. The more fat you have stored, the more leptin you should secrete. Our brains respond to increased leptin levels by producing feelings of fullness and reducing hunger. Insulin and leptin are related: When insulin is high and fat is stored, leptin is released.

For those with very low body fat, leptin levels will be low: The brain will receive this message and tell you, "I need to eat!" For those with excess weight, the leptin levels should technically be higher, telling the brain not to eat, as there is enough stored.

Sounds like a perfect system, but this system doesn't work the same way in PCOS. The reason is that, like insulin resistance, women with PCOS are also prone to leptin resistance. Our brains no longer respond to the message that we have enough stored fat, and our appetite isn't suppressed by high levels of leptin. As a result, more food is consumed and more insulin is secreted, creating a vicious cycle.

In fact, women with PCOS, whether they are lean or carry extra weight, secrete more leptin than women without PCOS.[1] All of the excessive leptin we have floating around in our bodies desensitizes our brain, totally overriding the body's natural hunger mechanisms. To make it simple, when you are leptin resistant, your brain thinks you are starving and tells your body that it needs to store more fat.

Leptin resistance acts on your brain in the exact same way that low leptin levels do. It sends the message that you don't have enough stored fat for times when there isn't enough food. Leptin resistance makes you hungry, primarily for the foods that are the fastest form of energy or the most dense in calories, namely sugar or carbohydrates.

And so the cycle continues. To make matters worse, leptin resistance also lowers your metabolism, so that your body conserves energy and burns fewer calories.

Leptin resistance has been linked to inflammation of the hypothalamus—the same area of the brain that regulates our hormonal function. High leptin levels inhibit follicle-stimulating hormone (FSH), and this causes poor follicle development and stalls ovulation.

Adiponectin

Women with PCOS also have low levels of a protein called adiponectin. Adiponectin is secreted only by the fat cells, just like leptin is. Adiponectin is different than leptin, however. With leptin, the more fat cells you have, the more you secrete.

Adiponectin is the exact opposite: The more lean you are, the more you secrete. In fact, low levels of adiponectin are specifically found in people who have more visceral (abdominal) fat, which is the type of fat that many women with PCOS tend to have in excess.

Low levels of adiponectin predispose women with PCOS to more inflammation. Adiponectin also helps with insulin sensitivity: When there's not enough, it results in insulin resistance. Also, low adiponectin is associated with fatty liver disease, which is a common phenomenon found in PCOS. Adiponectin can be tested through many laboratories. It has been found that young girls who develop PCOS later have low adiponectin levels during childhood. In fact, even in young and lean women, it has been found that those with PCOS were 3.2 times more likely to have lower adiponectin levels.

Insulin Resistance

When we have the chronic low-grade inflammation that goes along with PCOS (or even more so with having the excess abdominal fat deposition with PCOS), our cells become insulin resistant. Women with PCOS are much more prone to insulin resistance than others, due in part to genetics and increased baseline inflammation.

In insulin resistance, the cells don't respond to the message of insulin after eating, and too much sugar remains in the blood and doesn't get taken up into the cells. The pancreas senses this high blood sugar and sends out even more insulin to drive the sugar into the cells and keep the blood sugar under control. This causes an overall increased baseline level of insulin in the bloodstream, which is out of proportion to the blood sugar level at any given time. High insulin levels aggravate your ovaries, causing them to produce androgens like testosterone, and generally cause problems with many of the tissues in your body. The oxidative stress and inflammation caused by insulin resistance disrupt the way that your body functions.

Some common physical signs of insulin resistance include the deposition of fat around the waist, difficulty losing weight, dark, velvety pigmentation in the folds of skin behind the neck or under the arms (acanthosis nigricans), and the formation of skin tags.

Diabetes

Most women with PCOS don't have diabetes, but they are at risk. Insulin resistance, over time, causes the pancreas to have to increase its output of insulin to compensate for the unmanaged blood sugar. High blood sugar is very damaging to our cells, but particularly to the cells in our pancreas. The pancreas will produce insulin for as long as it can, but eventually it will give out, and the cells will begin to die. In addition, it's thought that lipotoxicity also affects the pancreas. Inflammatory damage is involved in the development of type 2 diabetes in women with PCOS.

When the pancreatic cells die, they can no longer produce the insulin needed to control the blood sugar. As a result, our blood sugar levels rise, causing type 2 diabetes. If you are at risk, you will want to pay special attention to the section on treatments for insulin resistance later in this chapter. For now, know that insulin resistance on its own is very damaging to your body.

Hypoglycemia

Women with PCOS often have ups and downs in blood sugar. This is a direct result of insulin resistance. Since insulin levels are high, our bodies can also pull too much sugar out of the bloodstream at any given time, causing a "sugar crash," leaving us shaky, hungry, and irritable. The more carbohydrates you consume, the more your insulin will spike, and the harder you will crash as your blood sugar drops. It's been found that women with PCOS are more prone to reactive hypoglycemia, where the blood sugar drops abruptly within two to five hours after a meal. Evidence shows that the women with the most marked reactive hypoglycemia were also the ones most prone to insulin resistance.[2]

High insulin levels also reduce the secretion of a hormone known as glucagon, which, although it sounds similar, is different than glycogen. Glucagon is released when our blood sugar drops, and it helps us to release the energy in stored fat or glycogen to keep blood sugar regulated. When insulin is high, glucagon can't do its job. As such, we can experience drops in blood sugar and much less burning of fat between our mealtimes, when we have insulin resistance.

Cortisol

To learn more about cortisol, please read the chapter on the adrenals. For now, know that women with PCOS have been found to have high levels of the stress hormone cortisol compared to women without PCOS.

Cortisol plays a key role when it comes to blood sugar regulation. When blood sugar drops, our body perceives this as a stress. Cortisol is then released by the adrenal glands, telling the body to burn glycogen or fat and increase blood sugar levels. Cortisol also increases insulin resistance. It decreases the uptake of glucose from the bloodstream and increases its breakdown in the liver. This increases blood glucose levels overall, which means that even more insulin is needed to manage the situation. In addition to increasing insulin resistance, cortisol also directs fat storage to the abdominal region—the area that is the absolute worst when it comes to insulin resistance, and the exact area that is a major aggravating factor for women with PCOS.

Stress and cortisol make insulin resistance worse and feed into the hormonal cycle that disrupts our metabolisms. For more information on the adrenal glands, please see chapter 4.

Androgens

High levels of insulin cause the ovaries to make too much testosterone. As we've learned, increased androgens are a central factor in PCOS: They stall ovulation and create hirsutism, acne, and hair loss. When the body is resistant to insulin, the ovaries remain sensitive to its effects, and they respond to increased levels of insulin by secreting plenty of androgens.

Interestingly, there are some women who have "hidden" PCOS. When they gain weight and their insulin levels rise, they will start producing androgens, and their PCOS will become uncovered. At a lower weight, or in a less insulin resistant condition, their PCOS symptoms will be reversed.

Insulin Resistance Testing

Measuring your glucose levels alone means relatively nothing with respect to insulin resistance. You can have completely normal blood sugar and yet have insulin resistance. Why? Insulin resistance is not diabetes and is present for years before it develops. So, how do you actually test for insulin resistance if typical diabetes testing isn't going to pick it up? Here are some tips.

Fasting Insulin and Fasting Glucose

After a minimum of ten hours of fasting, a ratio between fasting insulin and glucose, called the *HOMA-IR*, can be calculated, which provides a measure of insulin resistance. Elevated fasting glucose is a marker of diabetes, but it is often normal in insulin resistance. I always aim for a fasting insulin level below 50 pmol/L (under 7 uIU/mL) in my patients and a HOMA-IR of under 1.0.

Insulin-Glucose Challenge Test

This more sensitive test can pick up insulin resistance at its earliest stages. You drink a quantity of glucose and measurements of both insulin and glucose are taken over two or four hours. This test can detect early stages of insulin resistance, even when fasting insulin and blood glucose markers are totally normal.

HBA1C

This is a test that measures your average blood glucose over two to three months. Typically, any level below 5.6 is considered normal. Levels from 5.6 to 6.4 indicate that prediabetes may exist. Above this, diabetes is likely.

Treatments for Insulin Resistance in PCOS

The number one most effective treatment for treating insulin resistance in PCOS is regulating diet and exercise. I cannot emphasis enough how your life will be transformed simply by changing the foods that you eat and by exercising. No supplement or medication listed here will ever come close to bringing you the benefits you'll get from making those simple lifestyle changes. For more information on diet, be sure to read chapter 9, which goes into detail for those interested in a unique insulin-counting and anti-inflammatory nutritional approach to help restore normal insulin signaling in your body. By changing our diets, we can manage the amount of insulin we secrete.

Insulin Resistance and Weight Loss—A Different Outlook for Women with PCOS

The first thing most women with PCOS hear when they go to the doctor for help is "if you could just lose x number of pounds, you'd feel better." For women with lifelong weight struggles, if there were an easy way to "just lose weight," they would already have done so! The fact is it's not that simple, particularly when it comes to PCOS.

As a general rule, what you weigh is not a choice, but rather, a function of genetics, hormones, and neurotransmitters and is greatly affected by your childhood weight and the way that food is viewed culturally and within our families.

Once we have been at a certain weight for a significant amount of time, studies show that dieting causes initial weight loss followed by regain (often with additional weight tacked on top). When a person is heavy for a number of years, or particularly from childhood, their metabolism works very differently from that of a person who has always been lean. It is much more difficult for a person of significant size to lose weight and then maintain that weight than it is for someone who has always been lean to maintain that very same weight.

When a person is insulin resistant, the brain creates a new "normal" set point: It wants to hold onto its fat stores, and for every pound that is lost, metabolism slows down in an attempt to regain any lost body mass. Thyroid hormones drop, cell metabolism slows, appetite increases, and fat is stored with more efficiency for every lost pound. Our bodies have an amazing capacity to survive times when there isn't enough food, and this is that very mechanism in action. As a result, most diets cause cycles of weight loss and then regain, ultimately damaging the metabolism even more. This is true for all people, but is particularly true for women with PCOS.

As such, I believe that focusing on weight loss is an ineffective way to address PCOS-related insulin resistance. In fact, research shows that despite the widespread belief that a high body mass index is unhealthy, there are large percentages of people in the high BMI category who are in fact very healthy, with excellent cardiometabolic bloodwork profiles.[3] I can't tell you the number of women in my practice who technically have a high body mass index, follow an excellent program of nutrition and exercise, and their bloodwork indicates nothing but great health. Despite this, they continue to feel judged by health-care professionals, or sadly are even accused about being untruthful about their lifestyle and nutritional habits and are told they must eat less. We really need to see a change in medicine to reflect what we now know about metabolic health, and it needs to happen soon!

Rather than restrictive dieting, focusing on insulin resistance through a nutritional method, such as the one outlined in chapter 9, is often very successful. Most women who are insulin resistant will lose weight with this method, but it will occur only as the result of a healthier metabolism. The weight lost while you are eating healthfully, exercising, and managing your insulin resistance may eventually take you to your recommended "body mass index" level. However, it may not, and that is totally fine. You can achieve your personal best health at any size.

It is far better to achieve a healthy, natural, and stable weight based on a foundation of good nutrition than it is to swing back and forth between high and low weights. Putting women through diets that ultimately do more harm than good and cause more weight gain in the end just doesn't make sense.

In addition to all of this, dieting can trigger bingeing and other eating disorders, which women with PCOS are already prone to. They also cause you to ignore your natural hunger and fullness cues. When we are trying to cultivate good responses between the brain and metabolic hormones, restrictive dieting only takes us farther away from our ultimate goals.

Exercise

As exercise directly reduces insulin resistance, it's a key helper in minimizing inflammation for women with PCOS. For women who have increased abdominal fat stores, implementing an exercise program can absolutely be a game changer.

It doesn't have to be a huge amount of exercise, either. Studies have found that just seventy-five minutes per week of vigorous exercise, like jogging, high-intensity interval training, or vigorous swimming, can significantly improve metabolic health for women with PCOS.[4]

I recommend starting with this seventy-five minutes weekly as a baseline and then going up from there. Exercise can improve the physical aspects of PCOS, like inflammation and insulin resistance. But more than that, it can help with self-confidence and mood—something that many women with PCOS have challenges with due to the distressing symptoms of the condition. If you enjoy the benefits of exercise, see if you can find a dedicated personal trainer who understands PCOS and insulin resistance to help take you to the next level.

Conventional Medical Treatment for Insulin Resistance

Metformin

This is the most commonly used pharmaceutical drug for the treatment of insulin resistance in women with PCOS. It's even been called vitamin M due to its widespread application. I don't call it that, but I also don't dispute that it can be helpful for many women. However, my goal is to get your body's hormones working to the point that you don't need strong medications to alter its function. If your insulin, leptin, and glucose signaling pathways work, the vast majority of women *can* reverse insulin resistance and eliminate the need to take any of the pharmaceutical treatments listed here.

Metformin is often prescribed for women with PCOS, whether they are lean or larger-sized. For those who are trying to conceive, it's often combined with fertility drugs. That being said, there is a rather large subset of lean women for whom it has little to no effect. Given that it works primarily on insulin resistance, this makes complete sense. I've also found through clinical practice that in lean women with PCOS, who have very minimal insulin resistance, it doesn't seem to provide much benefit.

Metformin works in part by affecting the action of the mitochondria, which are like the batteries of our cells. This effect is very strong in the liver, decreasing the liver's output of glucose. This reduces the oxidation of fatty acids (lipotoxicity) and increases the uptake of glucose in our tissues. Metformin can lower fasting insulin levels without lowering blood sugar.

But there are the long-lamented side effects. A large percentage of women will experience these, and for many women, these are completely intolerable. The side effects consist of nausea, diarrhea, vomiting, bloating, and abdominal discomfort. In fact, when compared to placebo, metformin causes a fourfold increase in abdominal symptoms. Often, metformin is gradually increased to minimize these side effects: Typical doses range from 500 mg to 2,000 mg.

Metformin also affects the microbiome (the community of bacteria) in the gastrointestinal (GI) tract profoundly, and it is thought that this is, in part, how it affects metabolism. Metformin shifts the type of bacteria that reside in the intestinal area toward bacteria that seem to promote improvements in metabolism. After treatment with metformin, the bacteria in the gut produce more anti-inflammatory products, such as butyrate and short chain fatty acids—all of which have been associated with improvements in metabolism.[5]

A rare but serious complication of metformin is lactic acidosis. This condition has a fatality rate of up to fifty percent. In addition, metformin can decrease your uptake of vitamin B12. As such, all women on this medication should be taking 1,000 mcg of methylcobalamin (active B12).

In addition to its effects on the mitochondria, it has also been found that metformin can affect something called one-carbon metabolism, or methylation.[6] This is a hugely important factor in DNA repair and cell division, and it may be in part how it works to reduce the growth of cancer cells, as metformin has also been used to treat cancer patients. That being said, one carbon metabolism is also very important when it comes to fertility and pregnancy, where cell growth occurs at a rapid rate.

As a result, some researchers are very concerned about the long-term possible effects of metformin on the fetus—particularly when used in women who are not insulin resistant, where the benefit may not outweigh the potential risks.

Several short-term studies on metformin have associated it with a reduction in miscarriage rate and gestational diabetes in insulin-resistant women with PCOS, with no increase in major birth defects. Unfortunately, there are no long-term studies following the outcomes in babies whose mothers took metformin in pregnancy, so as of now its safety during pregnancy is unknown.

Natural Medicines for Insulin Resistance

The Inositols

Inositol is perhaps one of the most researched supplements for PCOS. There are two major forms of inositol. Myo-inositol is a sugar alcohol that is a relative of the B vitamin family, while D-chiro-inositol is what is known as a chiral epimer of myo-inositol. Simply put, they have a similar shape, just like your two hands do, but they do not match when you place one over the other, as shown in Figures 3-2 and 3-3.

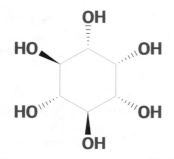

Figure 3-2: Myo Inositol

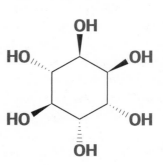

Figure 3-3: D-Chiro-Inositol

In addition, the different forms of inositol improve insulin sensitivity, correcting the hormonal system in PCOS and promoting healthy ovulation. Some of the actions of insulin are, in fact, mediated by inositol, and researchers have found that women with PCOS may have defects in inositol-insulin signaling pathways that are involved in insulin resistance. As such, myo-inositol has been classified as an insulin-sensitizing agent and is one of the most commonly used natural therapeutics for PCOS.[7] Typical doses for myo-inositol range from 2,000 to 4,000 mg per day.

D-Chiro-Inositol

D-chiro-inositol is made from myo-inositol, and research has found that women with PCOS excrete six times more D-chiro-inositol (DCI) than women without the condition.[8] Research suggests that the more DCI that is excreted, the more insulin resistance the patient will have. One study concluded that the excretion of excessive amounts of DCI may actually be a central factor in the insulin resistance of PCOS. D-chiro-inositol is not found readily in food like myo-inositol. Typical doses range from 100 mg to 600 mg per day. For information specific to fertility and the different forms of inositol, please see Appendix A.

It is important not to "overdose" on DCI. However, at the right dose, it can assist with egg and embryo quality in women with insulin-resistant PCOS. On occasion, inositol can cause mild side effects. These are rare and may include loose stools and stomach upset.

Berberine

One of the most effective supplements for PCOS insulin resistance, berberine has long been used for the treatment of diabetes in the realm of traditional Chinese medicine. It is an insulin sensitizer sharing some of the same mechanisms with the same level of efficacy as, or potentially even better than, metformin.[9] Not surprisingly, it tends to produce similar changes in the GI microbiome as the metformin. However, it boasts a much better side effect profile with not nearly the same amount of GI side effects. Berberine is not systemically absorbed as much as metformin is and actually may exert more of its beneficial impact on the microbiome rather than the mitochondria and other cellular functions. Not surprisingly, given the effect on the microbiome, it also has an excellent anti-inflammatory profile and has been found to reduce many of the inflammatory mediators, such as NF-kappa B and TNF-alpha. A study on eighty-nine insulin-resistant women with PCOS found that 500 mg three times per day significantly improved metabolic markers of insulin resistance, such as HOMA-IR,[10] even better than metformin did. Since berberine is a natural agent that has the same level of efficacy as a pharmaceutical, its use should be closely monitored. Berberine does have several important drug interactions, particularly with the macrolide antibiotics azithromycin and clarithromycin. As such, I recommend its use under the supervision of a physician or naturopathic physician. When used properly, however, it may be more effective than metformin for the management of insulin resistance with fewer side effects and other benefits, including a reduction of total and LDL cholesterol, triglycerides, HbA1c (a marker of diabetes), and inflammatory markers.

Resveratrol

This compound found in the skin of grapes has shown promise for both PCOS and for insulin resistance. Multiple animal studies have shown that it can reduce the overproliferation of the ovarian theca cells that are the cause of excess androgen production.[11] However, another study showed that it wasn't as effective as exercise, showing once again that no supplement can match the benefits of diet and exercise for insulin resistance.[12] One benefit of resveratrol, as already discussed, is that it is also anti-inflammatory, which means it may help to mediate lipotoxicity and protect our tissues from damage. As mentioned in the chapter on inflammation, the trans form of resveratrol is the most effective at doses ranging from 100 to 250 mg per day.

Glucomannan

This is a soluble fiber extract that has a very thick and viscous texture. It slows down carbohydrate absorption and can dampen the insulin response after a meal up to fifty percent.[13] It has some benefits for weight loss and promotes feelings of fullness after eating. I use glucomannan in my practice quite often. Patients often note an initial adjustment period with this, as the increase in fiber can cause some loose stools or bloating. After several days, this symptom almost always stops. Glucomannan is a very safe therapeutic for women with PCOS who would like to reduce appetite and improve insulin sensitivity. Doses typically range from 1 to 2.5 grams per meal, always taken with a large glass of water.

Grape Seed Extract

Similar to resveratrol, grape seed extract is an anti-inflammatory supplement that can improve insulin sensitivity.[14] It can reduce lipotoxicity and has also been found to have a positive long-term effect on glucose regulation, as well as improving insulin resistance. Typical dosages of grape seed extract range from 50 to 100 mg per day.

Vitamin D

I don't want to overstate how important vitamin D is, but for women with PCOS, it's crucial to their health. Low vitamin D has been directly associated with insulin resistance, so it's important to make sure you are in the optimal zone with your levels.

Chromium

Chromium is a mineral that has long been used to treat insulin resistance. People who are deficient in chromium have an increased tendency to develop insulin resistance, and replenishing this deficiency can help. Typical doses of chromium picolinate or chromium GTF, which are two excellent forms, range from 200 to 400 mcg per day.

Selenium

A recent study found 200 mcg per day of selenium to be beneficial for women with PCOS, as it improved insulin resistance and lowered triglycerides.[15] Of note, another study found that taking too much selenium can deplete chromium. As such, if you are taking selenium, it's important to be sure you taking it with chromium. A good multivitamin should have both nutrients included in sufficient amounts.

Alpha Lipoic Acid

Alpha lipoic acid is a special antioxidant that has been found to increase insulin sensitivity. It has the ability, like insulin, to stimulate glucose uptake and metabolism. It improves glutathione levels, increasing cellular function. It also affects the brain. It suppresses the action of an enzyme known as AMP-activated protein kinase (AMPK), which is one of the same enzymes metformin is thought to act primarily on. Its action on AMPK tells the brain that there's enough glucose in the blood currently, causing the brain to send the signal out to stop eating, which may be helpful for both weight loss and insulin resistance. One study found that 600 mg per day of alpha lipoic acid improved insulin sensitivity and increased ovulation rates.[16]

Cinnamon

A favorite supplement for insulin resistance, cinnamon, at the dose of 1.5 grams per day, has been found to improve menstrual cyclicity in women with PCOS and to significantly improve insulin sensitivity.[17] It is thought that cinnamon may work to regulate both insulin sensitivity as well as the expression of genes in fat cells.

Fenugreek

This seed has been studied for the treatment of insulin resistance in diabetics. It appears to have hypoglycemic and antioxidant effects. It may, in part, work by reducing lipotoxicity and minimizing insulin resistance through this pathway. It has also been studied in women with PCOS at a dose of 1.5 grams per day and has been shown to reduce the polycystic appearance of the ovaries.[18]

Chapter 4

STEP 3. BALANCE YOUR ADRENALS AND IMPROVE YOUR MOOD

Each person deserves a day away in which no problems are confronted, no solutions searched for. Each of us needs to withdraw from the cares which will not withdraw from us.

—MAYA ANGELOU

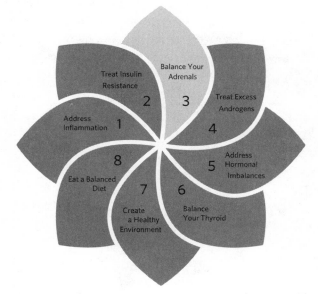

Gemma was a lawyer who worked on Bay Street in Toronto, the most fast-paced and competitive environment for a modern lawyer. Her days were typically fourteen to sixteen hours long, and she often worked late into the night, existing on shockingly little sleep. Then she would wake up each morning and do it all over again. Gemma also had PCOS, a condition she didn't know too much about, though she had been diagnosed with it at a young age. Except for her somewhat irregular periods and acne, it didn't bother her too much. Gemma, however, was completely stressed out.

She was often anxious and frequently woke up at night, worrying about the cases she was working on. She also had fatigue on many days and found it difficult to get through the afternoon without a serious crash. She would try to increase her energy by eating something sweet, perhaps a chocolate bar or a muffin. She was lean framed, so she never really worried about her sugar intake. These sugar fixes would help her energy temporarily, but soon enough she would crash once again. The other lawyers in the firm didn't seem to be as affected energy-wise as Gemma and certainly didn't seem as anxious. Could PCOS be the reason?

A Brief History of the Adrenal Glands

The adrenals are two triangular-shaped glands that sit above the kidneys. The adrenals secrete hormones in response to stress. The outer part of the adrenal gland, the cortex, makes cortisol and androgens like DHEA. In fact, a lot of androgens are produced in complex pathways in the adrenals. Cortisol is a very important hormone for our bodies. It's used to help us to handle stresses in the environment by increasing our blood sugar, suppressing the immune system, aiding in metabolism, and reducing bone formation. Cortisol shuts down many functions in the body that are not important to prioritize when we are in a stressful situation, making energy available for things like running away from predators that are chasing us.

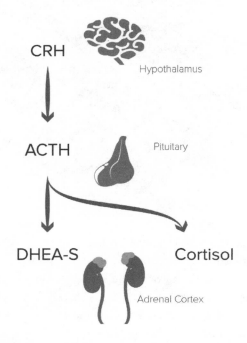

Figure 4-1: Adrenal Hormone Regulation

Like many of the other hormones in the body, the hypothalamus in the brain controls the release of cortisol. When stress is encountered in the environment, the hypothalamus makes corticotrophin-releasing hormone (CRH). CRH then signals the pituitary gland to make another hormone, adrenocorticotropic hormone (ACTH), which goes directly to the adrenal gland to do its work. Then the adrenal gland will make cortisol and DHEA, androgens that many women who have PCOS have elevated levels of.

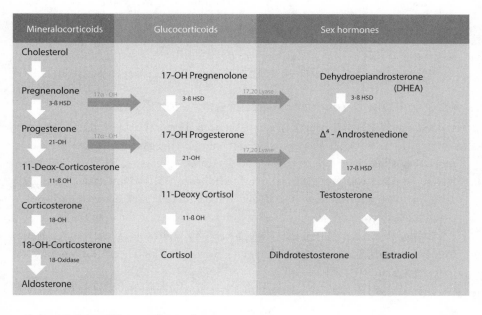

Figure 4-2: Adrenal Hormone Production

The Adrenals and Androgens

Some patients have an excess of androgens from their ovaries, and others from their adrenal glands. This leads to different "adrenal dominant" and "ovary dominant" androgen excess types. The topic of androgen excess in general, including ovarian androgens, is covered in the next chapter. Patients who are adrenal dominant tend to have less severe metabolic/cardiovascular risks than those who are ovary dominant, according to research.[1] This might be partly due to the fact that DHEA is a hormone that has many anti-aging and anti-inflammatory qualities. As such, it may provide some benefits that women who are more ovary androgen dominant are not getting. The other factor to consider is that often women who produce a lot of adrenal androgens are less insulin resistant, as DHEA is associated with lower insulin levels. Insulin resistance causes the ovary to make more testosterone. More androgens coming from the ovary can be a sign of insulin resistance itself.

It's not all good though. Adrenal androgens can still cause significant hormonal disruption in women, such as hirsutism, acne, hair loss, and the cessation of ovulation altogether. Around fifty percent of women with PCOS have significant amounts of androgens that originate from the adrenal glands.

When we are developing as embryos, our adrenals and ovaries actually develop from a similar tissue. As such, they have very similar enzymes within them. This is why many women with PCOS make androgens from their adrenal glands in addition to their ovaries. Researchers are still trying to identify the mechanisms. However, it seems that the androgens produced from the adrenals increase the androgen production from the ovaries and vice versa. It's a vicious cycle of androgens all around!

How to Know if You Have Adrenal Androgen Excess

Women can find out if they have an adrenal androgen excess by having their DHEA-S levels tested, as this androgen is made only by the adrenal glands. DHEA-S is a hormone that is high when we are young and decreases with age. As such, you need to look at DHEA-S with respect to your age (see Figure 4-3) and not at the reference range included with the test. If in doubt, you can ask an experienced health-care practitioner to compare your test result with what is average for your age range. If it is higher than average, you may have the adrenal androgen factor. Another way to identify if you have an adrenal androgen factor is to look at the ratio between testosterone and DHEA-S.

Typically, if the ratio is greater than 4.4, you may have more of an "adrenal" androgen type of PCOS. That being said, even if your ratio is not more than 4.4 and you have an elevated level of DHEA-S for your age, you likely have an adrenal androgen factor, where a significant amount of the androgens come from the adrenal glands rather than from the ovaries.

Research has found that young girls whose adrenals begin to activate earlier are at higher risk of PCOS. As girls mature, one of the first thing that happens, even before puberty, is the activation of the adrenals, which is known as adrenarche. Adrenarche occurs when the adrenals begin to secrete DHEA, which causes pubic hair and body hair to begin growing. Girls who get body hair early may have an increased risk for PCOS, as their adrenals are activating early. This has been associated with increased adrenal androgen formation throughout life.

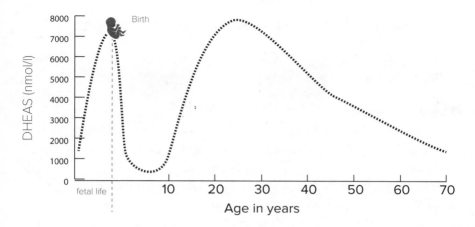

Figure 4-3: DHEA-S with Respect to Age

What Causes Us to Produce More Androgens from Our Adrenals

The main stimulator for the production of adrenal androgens (primarily DHEA) is stress. A hormone known as ACTH is produced by the pituitary gland in response to stress. ACTH causes the adrenals to make more DHEA. The excess DHEA is then converted into androgens by the adrenal glands.

As such, stress is absolutely the worst thing for women with an "adrenal androgen" factor. This is why women with adrenal androgen excess often benefit most from stress-relieving techniques and therapies.

PCOS and Cortisol

Another main hormone produced by the adrenal glands, and which is highly relevant to women with PCOS, is cortisol. Cortisol, as mentioned earlier, is our main stress hormone. Women with PCOS actually make *more* cortisol than women without PCOS. This happens as a result of complex enzymatic pathways in the adrenal glands that are upregulated, in similar ways to how our pathways that make androgens are upregulated. Over time, if a woman with PCOS endures a great deal of stress, her adrenals will produce more cortisol than average, and this is a continuous strain on the adrenal glands themselves.

Interestingly, a study found that lean women with PCOS made more cortisol than the lean control group.[2] This is significant, because when a person is overweight, they often produce more cortisol. As such, studying lean women identified only the difference in cortisol caused by having PCOS, rather than any difference in weight. So, although it's true that having PCOS increases cortisol, being heavy, which is a common tendency in PCOS, increases it further. So, many women with PCOS have a double whammy when it comes to too much cortisol.

Thus, we can truly say that there is a physiological reason that stress is actually more aggravating to us, and we must find ways to manage it.

Cortisol and Progesterone

As we'll learn in chapter 6, progesterone is a hormone that is often severely deficient in women with PCOS. As ovulation may not be timed well and is often not produced at all, less progesterone is available to balance out the cycle.

In the adrenals, cortisol is made from progesterone and its precursor, pregnenolone. When the hypothalamic pituitary adrenal axis is stimulated, cortisol levels are high and there is an acute increase in hormone production. This occurs particularly along the adrenal androgen branch, and DHEA then converts these hormones into testosterone.

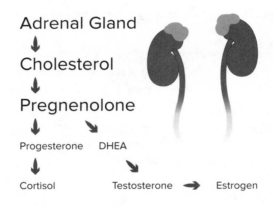

Figure 4-4: Adrenal-Progesterone

However, after prolonged periods of stress and chronically high cortisol levels, hormone production on the whole decreases, and you'll see a reduction the body's ability to manufacture both cortisol and all other hormones, particularly the female hormones, including both estrogen and progesterone. This is also, at least in part, related to a decrease in leptin. This is typically called "hypothalamic amenorrhea." In some instances, I have noted that certain women with PCOS can experience hypothalamic amenorrhea when highly stressed, with rapid weight loss or extremely intense exercise (especially in lean PCOS), or after stopping the birth control pill. Stress can therefore make many of the hormonal aspects of PCOS much worse.

Cortisol and Other Hormones

Your hormones become less effective when cortisol levels are high. This is because high levels of cortisol cause abnormalities in the way that many of the sex hormones and thyroid hormones work in the body. Raised cortisol levels make the cells in your body less able to use estrogen, progesterone, and thyroid hormones, and also reduce the conversion of the inactive form of thyroid hormone T4 into the active form of thyroid hormone T3. You will learn more about this in chapter 7, when we explore how to balance thyroid dysfunction.

As thyroid dysfunction is more common in PCOS, this can really aggravate your condition. High cortisol also reduces the cellular sensitivity to thyroid hormone. Basically, stress makes all of the hormones work in a less effective way.

Adrenal Fatigue vs. Adrenal Hyperactivity

First, it's important to know what our adrenal glands are supposed to do throughout a typical day. Cortisol helps us wake up in the morning. It should rise when we rise, giving us energy to begin our day. After that point, it naturally decreases and reaches its lowest point in the evening hours, as shown in Figure 4-5. Any sort of stress, such as emotional stress, low blood sugar, or physical stress, can increase the cortisol at any given time.

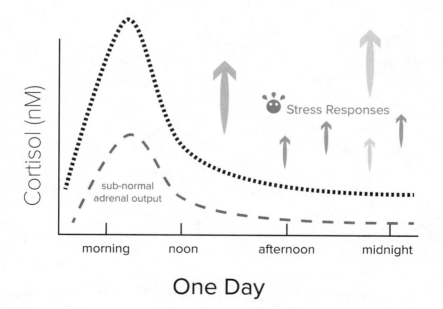

Figure 4-5: Circadian Cortisol Rhythm

The following can be indicative of hyperactive adrenal glands and high cortisol levels in the body:

- Weight gain around the stomach
- Anxiety
- Insomnia
- Suppressed immune system
- Wired and tired feeling
- Irritability
- Increased blood sugar
- Insulin resistance

You may have heard of the term "adrenal fatigue." It indicates that a person has experienced so much stress, whether physical or emotional, and has secreted so much cortisol over time that their adrenals can no longer keep up with the body's demands. In people who have adrenal fatigue, you'll see that their cortisol curve is abnormal, and that their cortisol levels are typically lower than average.

Symptoms of adrenal fatigue include the following:

- Fatigue
- Depression
- Afternoon dip in energy
- Autoimmune disease
- Intense salt cravings
- Feeling better in the evening
- Dizziness
- Low blood pressure
- Frequent urination
- Low libido
- Hypoglycemia

Other women with PCOS can have high cortisol levels at different times during the day. This is considered a sort of adrenal hyperactivity. Women with PCOS can have either adrenal fatigue or adrenal hyperactivity or a combination of high and low cortisol at different times of the day. As such, many women may benefit from completing a salivary cortisol test to determine what sort of dysregulation may be happening in their adrenal glands that could be contributing to their PCOS.

Cortisol and Blood Sugar Regulation

As we know already, women with PCOS typically have insulin resistance as a key component. To make matters worse, high cortisol also causes insulin resistance. After a stressful event and an elevation in cortisol, insulin resistance develops after four to six hours and persists for more than sixteen hours.[3] Stress can make your metabolic health worse, and as we know, insulin resistance delays ovulation, causes excess androgens to be produced, and increases fat storage, which are all bad things for PCOS. It's important to know there are some women with PCOS who have adrenal fatigue. Although typically this is associated with hypoglycemia, it is still possible for insulin resistance to be present due to the overlying metabolic issues from PCOS.

PCOS, Anxiety, and Depression

Let's talk about something really important for women with PCOS: anxiety and depression. These conditions are rampant in our community, and for good reason. PCOS is a stressful condition to have, and with its side effects of hirsutism, acne, weight gain, infertility, and irregular cycles, it is certainly no surprise that women with PCOS often struggle psychologically as well. Anxiety and depression are associated with changes in cortisol.

In addition, emotional disorders have been linked to having high levels of androgens.[4] Even low-grade inflammation, the type of inflammation common in PCOS, has been linked to mood disorders like depression. Overall, it's quite clear why there is a prevalence of depression and anxiety in women with PCOS.

A recent meta-analysis of twenty-eight studies following over five thousand women found consistently higher levels of emotional distress in women with PCOS when compared to controls.[5] This study found that, in particular, women with medical "obesity" and hirsutism were more at risk for depression and anxiety overall. However, when analyzed, these factors did not fully account for the associations between PCOS and emotional distress. The study found that depression was present in women who were lean and fertile and in women who were considered "obese and infertile," leading the researchers to suggest there was another factor at play—a factor outside of those that are normally considered by society to be stressful. The researchers thought that perhaps inflammation or testosterone might be causing these imbalances.

In any case, knowing that these factors are more of a risk, we need to watch ourselves and care for ourselves in times of stress to ensure that we are not becoming "dis-stressed."

As we discussed in chapter 4, the hypothalamic pituitary axis is quite sensitive to stress and mood. Our hormones often alter when our brains perceive stress. The opposite is also true: Our brains can adapt in response to changes in hormones like cortisol. As such, we need to look at the mind-body connection closely in PCOS, if we are to achieve our best balance.

Treatments for Adrenal Conditions

There are different ways we can improve the health of our adrenals, ranging from lifestyle changes to nutrition. It's essential to address the underlying causes of increased stress, such as difficulty sleeping, emotional stressors, or increased family or work pressure.

Adrenal Androgens

Many of the treatments for adrenal androgen excess are quite similar to those found in the chapter on androgens. In addition, knowing that stress can increase the production of DHEA from the adrenals, through increasing ACTH, treating stress is directly helpful. When it comes to treating adrenal androgens, we want to focus on the ACTH responses that increase DHEA production within the adrenal glands.

Fish Oil and Omega-3 Fatty Acids

The omega-3 fatty acids found in fish oil may have a significant effect on blunting adrenal responses to stress, according to research.[6] In addition, multiple studies have found that fish oils and omega-3 fatty acids improve mood, with benefits ranging from reducing anxiety to alleviating depression. Typical doses of fish oil range from 1,000 to 3,000 mg per day. See chapter 2 for information on the amount of eicosapentaenoic acid (EPA) to aim for in your fish oil.

L-Theanine

L-theanine is an amino acid found in abundance in tea. This amino acid has been used widely for its calming effects and for promoting mental alertness. A recent study placed mice in a stressful territorial situation. Changes in the adrenal glands were studied in these mice, and it was found that the adrenal glands actually enlarged in size for the mice in the stressful living situation. The ingestion of theanine, however, significantly suppressed this overgrowth of the adrenal cells and normalized the secretion of ACTH in the blood. Typical doses of L-theanine range from 200 to 1000 mg per day.[7]

Phosphatidylserine

Phosphatidylserine is an important component of our cell membranes in that it helps our cells signal each other. As a supplement, it has benefits that can help to minimize the impact of stress on our adrenal glands. One study found that 200 mg of phosphatidylserine/phosphatidic acid complex per day may help to normalize ACTH and serum cortisol secretion in chronically stressed individuals.[8] Another study found that 800 mg of phosphatidylserine per day reduced stress-induced activation of the hypothalamic-pituitary-adrenal axis.[9]

Licorice

Glycyrrhiza glabra, commonly known as licorice, is an herb often used in formulas to tonify the adrenal glands. Licorice can slow the breakdown of adrenal hormones in the body and is helpful for women who have adrenal fatigue. In addition, 3.5 grams daily of a preparation of licorice (containing 7.6 percent glycyrrhizic acid) was found in a 2004 trial to significantly decrease testosterone levels in healthy female patients after one month of treatment.[10] The study concluded that licorice may exert its anti-androgenic action by blocking key enzymes involved in androgen production. It is important to note that licorice can increase blood pressure and shouldn't be used by women who have high blood pressure. In many cases, licorice is used as part of a combination formula, which is described in chapter 5.

Red Sage

Known as red sage, danshen, or Chinese sage, *Salvia miltiorrhiza* is a plant often used in traditional Chinese medicine. The root of danshen contains a substance known as cryptotanshinone, which has been shown to provide benefits for women with excess androgens originating from the adrenal glands. In a study on animals, rats were given PCOS through the injection of the adrenal androgen DHEA. The menstrual cycles of the animals given danshen improved significantly, and the adrenal androgen pathways were downregulated. It also improved testosterone, LH, SHBG, fasting insulin, and reduced the cystic appearance of the ovaries. Typical doses range from 200 mg to 1 gram daily.[11]

Vitex

Research suggests that high levels of prolactin are associated with rises in ACTH, 17-OHP, cortisol, and DHEA-S. Thus, if you suspect that you may have high prolactin (if you've had it in the past for example), *Vitex agnus-castus* may be a good herb for helping improve adrenal function. Lowering prolactin levels can actually decrease the production of androgens from the adrenals. In addition, vitex has well-known benefits for mood. It's been found to be effective in reducing irritability, depressed mood, and anxiety. A thorough discussion of vitex, including dosage, is included in chapter 6.

St. John's Wort

Hypericum perforatum, also known as St. John's wort, is one of the most researched natural treatments for mild to moderate depression. It's been found to reduce stress-induced increases in plasma ACTH and cortisol levels. As such, it may be of great benefit for women with PCOS who have mood disorders like depression or anxiety. You should note, however, that St. John's wort interacts with a great number of medications and must be used with caution as a result. It can also increase the skin's sensitivity to the sun, so be mindful of that when taking it. The most common dose of St. John's wort is 300 mg, three times daily.[12]

Golden Root

Rhodiola is a plant that normally grows in the northern hemisphere and is resident in high altitude areas in the Arctic, Scandanavia, and other northern countries. *Rhodiola rosea*, commonly known as golden root, is a flowering plant that, when taken, has antidepressant effects and can improve fatigue. Overall, in the world of herbal medicine, it's considered to be an adaptogen.

Many active phytochemicals have been identified in *Rhodiola rosea* that are physiologically active. It's thought that these components work primarily by regulating the hypothalamic-pituitary-adrenal axis and controlling mediators of stress responses like cortisol. The main active ingredient in *Rhodiola*, salidroside, has been found to reduce the expression of corticotrophic-releasing hormone in the brain, significantly reducing levels of cortisol and regulating the hypothalamic-pituitary-adrenal axis. Some new information suggests that *Rhodiola* improves the function of different stress sensor proteins in the brain, preventing energy loss in times of stress. Thus, for a woman with PCOS who is susceptible to stress, *Rhodiola* may be a beneficial herb.

Rhodiola also has mood-enhancing benefits and appears to help in particular patients who are suffering from depression. If a woman with PCOS has a strong adrenal factor and also suffers from depressive symptoms, *Rhodiola* is one of my favorite herbs to use. Doses of *Rhodiola* typically range from 50 to 600 mg per day.

Holy Basil

Holy basil, also known as tulsi (*Ocimum tenuiflorum*), is a fragrant plant that is native to Southeast Asia. It's used commonly in Ayurvedic medicine and although it is a relative of basil, it is a completely different plant altogether. Holy basil exerts effects on adrenal function by lowering cortisol while benefiting blood sugar control.

Holy basil also may be a beneficial herb for women with PCOS who have stress. One important thing to note, just in case your partners are taking supplements along with you, is that holy basil is not recommended for those who are trying to conceive, as it contains ursolic acid, which is considered a contraceptive agent. Typical doses of holy basil range from 100 to 500 mg two times daily.

Vitamin C
Vitamin C, also known as ascorbic acid, is a crucial vitamin for the function of the adrenal glands. Vitamin C, when given to people under stress, can minimize the excessive production of cortisol and can alleviate inflammation, which are beneficial for women with PCOS. Typical doses of vitamin C for stress are around 1000 mg per day.

Melatonin
For women with PCOS who have trouble with their sleep, melatonin can help. A study found that taking melatonin could reduce the ACTH stimulation of the adrenal glands in those who were deficient in this sleep-promoting hormone. Typical doses of melatonin for sleep range from 1.5 to 3 mg at bedtime.

Siberian Ginseng
Also known as Siberian ginseng, *Eleutherococcus senticosus* is a popular adaptogen that improves energy and minimizes the impact of stress on the brain. It regulates the hypothalamic-pituitary-adrenal axis, improving performance in stressful situations. This is an excellent herb for women who are fatigued and facing increased levels of daily stress in their lives. Typical doses for Siberian ginseng range from 300 mg to 4 grams daily.

Five-Flavor Berry
Shisandra chinensis, or five-flavor berry, is an herb from traditional Chinese medicine that has been used for thousands of years for its antistress benefits. It's a calming herb, and a 2007 study backed this up, showing that it was an effective protector against stress-related increases in cortisol in animals.[14] In addition, *Schisandra* can be quite helpful for people who have stress-induced insomnia. Typical doses range from 500 mg to 2 grams daily.

Myo-Inositol
As great as myo-inositol is for ovulation and insulin resistance, it provides another important benefit: It helps to mitigate stress. Particularly at high doses, it can reduce

anxiety, so it's a great two-in-one supplement. For more on dosage, please see chapter 3 and Appendix A.

Magnesium

Magnesium is required for so many processes within the nervous and hormonal system, and low levels have been consistently found in people with insulin resistance. It has known calming effects and can mitigate stress. Several studies have found that magnesium, especially when used with other vitamins or herbs, can mitigate symptoms of anxiety. Many people find that bedtime is the best time of day to take magnesium as it promotes calm sleep.[15] Typical doses of magnesium range from 200 to 600 mg per day in the form of citrate, or glycinate.

B-Complex Vitamins

We all think of the B-complex vitamins as being essential for stress. This is for good reason. Vitamin B5, also known as pantothenic acid, is necessary for the production of coenzyme A, and its deficiency can result in adrenal insufficiency. Research has found that injecting stress hormones into people can decrease their levels of folate and vitamin B12. As such, these hormones are essential to replace if a patient is under a great deal of stress.

Vitamin B6 is known for its benefits for hormonal regulation, premenstrual syndrome, and improving progesterone levels. These are all issues that women with PCOS may suffer from. A good B complex is beneficial for women with PCOS who are going through significant levels of stress.

Cordyceps

Cordyceps militaris is a mushroom that has long been used to improve immunity and overall stress indices. In multiple studies, cordyceps has been found to improve stamina and reduce fatigue in times of stress for both animals and humans. It also appears to reduce blood sugars in diabetics and those with higher blood sugar levels. As such, for women who may suffer from low cortisol, poor energy, and stress, cordyceps can be a great addition for women with PCOS. Typical doses of corydyceps range from 500 mg to 3 grams daily.

Blood Sugar Control

Something I'd like to mention is that blood sugar control is very important when it comes to keeping the adrenal glands healthy. Each and every time that blood sugar levels drop, your levels of cortisol rise. As such, keeping healthy and balanced blood sugar is an important part of keeping your adrenals healthy and your androgens under control, which we explore further in the chapters on insulin resistance and diet. The effects of our diet go far beyond weight and deeply into our hormonal balance. The sections that follow offer ways to manage stress levels for optimum adrenal health.

Meditation, Mindfulness, Yoga, and Prayer

Numerous studies have identified the benefits of meditation and prayer on the stress parameters in the human body. For example, a study following twenty-seven volunteers doing meditation found significant improvements in daytime secretion of the pituitary hormones like ACTH.[16]

Another recent trial in 2015 followed thirty-eight women with PCOS on a mindfulness stress-management program.[17] It was found that the women in the program had significant improvements in cortisol levels, as well as symptoms of anxiety, depression, and stress. It's been substantiated in scientific literature that relaxation techniques like yoga, meditation, and prayer can have profound benefits on mood, depression, and anxiety for people with these disorders.[18]

Loving Connections and Social Friendships

As women with PCOS, it's easy to feel stigmatized by our differences. Hair growth in areas not deemed acceptable by society, acne, weight gain, and the other symptoms of PCOS can create low self-esteem and feelings of isolation. It's especially important for women who have PCOS to connect with others with the same condition and to seek out friendships and romantic relationships only with people who are supportive. There's a virtual plethora of online communities today for women with PCOS to connect with each other and to receive expert support on dealing with some of the emotional aspects of the disorder.

Self-Care and Self-Esteem

The symptoms of PCOS can profoundly affect our self-esteem and how we feel in our identity as women. We are taught since childhood that a woman's value, at least in part, comes from her fertility and femininity. PCOS and the impact of androgens and excess insulin on our bodies can affect these aspects of our being, and so it's easy to feel that something is inherently "wrong" with you. This is not the case. When humans existed in a more natural environment, women with PCOS genes were the thrivers and survivors. They were the ones who could reproduce and survive in times of fewer resources. Our current environment, with toxins and processed foods, requires that we adjust, but it doesn't mean that we are flawed or less than. Unfortunately, much of society doesn't know this, and many women with PCOS are left feeling that they are not good enough due to their differences in body shape, size, and hormones. When you don't feel worthwhile, important, and valuable, it can make practicing the self-care needed to support your health very, very difficult.

I remember feeling awful about myself when I was a teenager. I felt unfeminine and tomboyish. Never having much interest in makeup, hair, or my looks, I was completely awkward and never felt I measured up. I only thought about what I was interested in, which was music and science. Looking back, I would love to talk to that young woman and tell her that she was completely OK. As a young girl, my interests were different from what society deemed typical for a female of my age, and I saw that as a negative thing, but those differences have really shaped who I am today.

It may help to look at a picture of yourself as a very small child, around two years old, or even just to picture her in your mind. She was amazing, and she deserved love simply because she existed. She also had endless potential, the potential to love, to grow, and to create. It can help you to see your inherent value by remembering that you are still the same person inside of that little girl. Just as she did then, you now deserve the same love, and you also hold great potential.

PCOS and its effects on our body size, shape, and expression of feminine or masculine characteristics—they are really part of human diversity. Diversity gives us many gifts that move us forward and bring us to new levels of understanding. Given that women with PCOS make up fifteen percent of the female population, our unique characteristics are very prevalent overall, and in that way, very natural and normal. I urge you to take a deeper look at your own unique gifts and positive qualities as you walk your path to healing. You may find that characteristics like empathy, strength, focus, determination, intellect, originality, resilience, and other positive qualities have grown in you as a result of your PCOS. Let these be your new guide as you make this journey towards the best version of yourself, physically and emotionally.

Counseling and Psychology

A good counselor, life coach, or psychologist can be invaluable for a woman with PCOS. As much as society can bring us down, sometimes we need experts in our lives who can lift us up and remind us of our value. Time spent with a good therapist can really change the way we think and the way we process events in our lives. A trial on twelve teenage women with PCOS found that just over eight sessions of cognitive behavioral therapy (CBT) resulted in an average weight loss of eleven kg and improved symptoms of depression.[19]

I hope this chapter has helped emphasize the whole-body effect that stress hormones create. The responses of the brain to stress can increase the secretion of androgens from our adrenal glands, disrupting the rhythm of hormones like estrogen and progesterone that not only regulate our cycles but also have profound effects on our brain and mood. Examining your stressors and stress levels and finding ways to reduce them through relaxation, community, and self-care, and (most importantly) learning to practice self-love and acceptance are essential to healing on your journey with PCOS.

Chapter 5

STEP 4. TREAT EXCESS ANDROGENS

*When she was a child, my love carried a road map in her
hand the way other girls carried handkerchiefs.*

—ROMAN PAYNE, *THE WANDERESS*

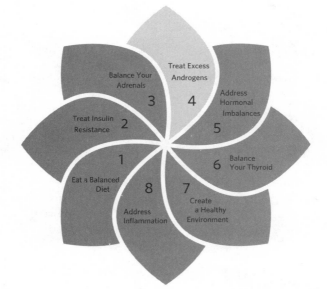

Cynthia was a twenty-eight-year-old woman who had been managing her PCOS for several years. Her periods were semiregular, showing up every thirty-five to forty days. What had really been bothering her, however, were the skin symptoms that often accompany a diagnosis of PCOS. Cynthia had been dealing with coarse hair growth on her chin and neck, known as hirsutism, which caused her a great deal of stress. No matter what she tried, it kept returning, and the amount seemed to be increasing over time.

In addition, she often broke out in inflammatory cystic acne that didn't seem to improve, despite the fact that she was well past her teenage years. She also noticed that her hair was beginning to thin. When she asked her doctor about these symptoms, she was told they were clearly related to PCOS. The excess testosterone produced by her ovaries was triggering all of these problems. She worked on her ovulatory function and began anti-androgenic natural medicine. Over time, she saw a significant change in all of the unwelcome androgen excess symptoms she had been experiencing.

Androgens in PCOS

Androgen excess in women has long been described in medical textbooks, dating back as early as 400 BC, with reports of women growing coarse hair in areas more commonly seen in men (such as the chin and upper lip), losing hair from the head, and in the manifestation of acne. High levels of hormones known as androgens (testosterone and similar hormones) are one of the most important diagnostic factors seen in women with PCOS and are even argued by some key researchers as being required for the diagnosis of PCOS.

There are a variety of different androgens to know about when it comes to your PCOS. These include—

- **Testosterone.** This is the most well-known androgen of all. It is derived approximately twenty-five percent from the adrenals, twenty-five percent from the ovaries, and fifty percent from the conversion of androstenedione in the bloodstream.
- **DHEA.** This is produced by the adrenals, and a small amount is also produced by the ovaries. DHEA pulses throughout the day in a similar way to cortisol.
- **DHEA-S.** This is the most abundant hormone in the circulation of women of reproductive age. It doesn't exhibit changes in its concentration throughout the day and is primarily produced by the adrenals.
- **Androstenedione.** This is a hormone that is produced fifty percent by the ovaries and fifty percent by the adrenals.
- **Dihydrotestosterone.** This is the most powerful androgen of all, and it is produced in the tissues of the body from testosterone.

Androgen Production

As young girls, we have similar levels of androgens to young boys. Adrenarche is the time in our young years before puberty when our adrenal glands first kick in and begin to produce hormones. When this happens, girls begin to produce pubic and underarm hair. It's thought that this process occurs because girls need to gain fat to prepare for their upcoming reproductive years. As such, the adrenals activate, releasing cortisol, which causes insulin resistance, helping the body to store fat more easily. When the adrenals secrete cortisol, as we've already learned, they also secrete the androgen DHEA-S. So, as girls go through this time, they tend to have a predominance of androgens.

Next, during typical puberty, when the female hormones start up, luteinizing hormone (LH) starts off as the predominant pituitary hormone. But as a girl begins to ovulate regularly, follicle-stimulating hormone (FSH) takes charge, bringing with it the all-important female hormone estrogen, which then takes center stage along with its sister hormone, progesterone.

It's now thought that perhaps PCOS is a hormonal state very similar to that of puberty, which hasn't fully completed, where LH, androgens, and insulin resistance are dominant, and the FSH, estrogen, and progesterone trio haven't been able to establish their full rhythm.[1] For a deeper look at these hormones, see chapter 6.

As puberty begins, and teenage girls approach their first ovulation, the ovaries also begin to produce testosterone. As a follicle that houses the egg goes through development in preparation for ovulation, it grows a variety of different supportive cells. The follicles contain two major types of hormone producing cells: the granulosa cells, which produce primarily estrogen, and the theca cells, which produce primarily testosterone. In women with PCOS, there is often an overproduction of testosterone by the theca cells in the ovary and even an overabundance of these cells overall. High levels of insulin stimulate the theca cells to grow and produce testosterone to an excessive degree.

Role of Androgens

Androgens are an essential part of every woman's health. They provide many vital functions, including improving our muscle mass, keeping our libido going strong, and moderating our body fat. They are necessary for bone, kidney, and liver health as well as fertility.

Too many androgens, however, now that's a different story. When these hormones are in excess, we can experience what is known as masculinization: Basically, when characteristics that are often thought of as "male" appear in women. These characteristics include hair growth in areas often seen in males and also acne, hair loss, and changes in body composition.

Hirsutism

Hirsutism (her-su-tism) is one of the most stressful and time-consuming problems experienced by women with PCOS. Hirsutism is the increase in hair growth in *specific* areas of the body, including the upper lip, chin, mid-chest, abdomen, and back. Excessive hair growth in other areas of the body, though bothersome, does not qualify as hirsutism.

PCOS is the most common cause of hirsutism, and it's thought that up to eighty-two percent of women with bothersome hair growth have PCOS. So, if someone you know is experiencing hirsutism, encourage them to have a checkup.

Blood Levels of Testosterone and Hirsutism

Although androgen excess underlies most cases of excessive hair growth, there is actually only a mild correlation between the levels of testosterone in the bloodstream and the growth of hair. In fact, it's mostly a concern that is related to the sensitivity of the hair follicle itself and a special enzyme called 5-alpha reductase. This enzyme converts testosterone to the more potent dihydrotestosterone or DHT.

There are two different types of 5-alpha reductase: Type 1 is found in the sebaceous glands (e.g., acne) and genital skin area, and Type 2 is found in the hair follicle and in the scalp. Type 2 activity is increased in disorders that have high levels of testosterone, like PCOS.

This increased activity causes problems with the hair follicle growth and prompts the hair to enter into the stage that causes it to soon fall out (telogen), which is what happens in alopecia. Once a hair enters telogen, it is preprogrammed to fall out within two to four months. Unfortunately, the opposite problem happens in the areas where hirsutism occurs. In this case, the hair follicle gets larger, wider, and stays in the growth phase longer. As you can tell, none of these are particularly good things when you are dealing with facial hair growth.

Insulin Resistance and 5-Alpha Reductase

The activity of 5-alpha reductase is also increased by insulin. Each woman with PCOS may experience a different level of excess hair growth, depending on her hair follicle sensitivity and insulin resistance levels.

When you notice that you have hirsutism, what should you do? Many women undergo androgen testing. Total testosterone is one of the most standard tests for women with hirsutism. Even so, the accuracy of this test is questionable. Despite obvious signs of high androgen levels, the majority of women with PCOS *have serum total testosterone levels within the normal range.*

Unfortunately, serum tests are not very good at picking up the presence of lower amounts of androgens, as are typically found in women (as compared to men who typically have much higher levels), so it is important not to place too much emphasis on whether or not your androgens are above the reference range on bloodwork. This does not matter, if you have symptoms of androgen excess, and it does not mean that anti-androgenic therapies will not work. They likely will. As mentioned earlier, the conversion in the skin and receptors may also be more involved, and these are difficult to measure through bloodwork.

DHT can be measured through the blood; however, like other androgens, the levels can be inaccurate. So, if you have hirsutism and your DHT is normal, you still may benefit from anti-androgen treatments.

DHEA and DHEA-S are adrenal androgens. When considering this, it is important to note that these hormones do decrease greatly with age. So, although reference ranges provided by the lab may be reliable in a younger woman, for an older woman, these levels should be ignored and should be assessed according to age instead.

Androgenetic Alopecia (Female-Pattern Hair Loss)

The loss of hair in women with PCOS is a hugely stressful aspect of the condition. I've seen women come to my office in tears more times than I can count over the loss of their hair. The hair-loss patterns in women with PCOS can vary from diffuse overall thinning of the hair and widening of the middle part, to thinning just behind the front hairline, and even to the sort of thinning at the temples that is seen in men. It's also the most common form of hair loss in women. It causes a reduction in the thickness of the hair, in addition to the loss of hair follicles and destruction of the follicles. This is something that affects fifty percent of all women in their lifetime, and it's characterized as a progressive loss of hair, meaning that it continues to fall out over time. It's well known that androgenetic alopecia is caused primarily by DHT and its effect on the hair follicle.

Of great importance to alopecia is what we call the "oxidative stress" that occurs at the level of the hair follicle when exposed to DHT. This oxidative stress is a big part of what results in the destruction of the follicle. Oxidative stress happens when different chemicals damage the cells. As discussed before, these chemicals can be produced during inflammation.

So not only do women with PCOS overproduce testosterone and have excessive inflammation, some also appear to have genetic alterations within the androgen receptor of the hair follicle itself. Not all women with PCOS will experience hair loss, so this may be why.

These special genes can be up- or downregulated by different things in the environment through a process known as epigenetics. Studies have found that there are actually increased amounts of androgen receptor genetic material in the hair follicles of the frontal scalp area for women with androgenetic alopecia.

In scalp hair follicles, the androgen receptor is a specific protein that DHT can bind to. Once DHT has bound, the receptor complex changes form, exposing the DNA binding sites of the hair cells.[2] This changes the way that the genes are expressed and causes the cells to die off in the follicle, resulting in hair loss.

Aromatase

Aromatase is an important enzyme to know about when it comes to androgens. It is present in different tissues, including the hair follicle. Aromatase can be a helper enzyme for women with PCOS. It converts testosterone to estrogen, which is often low. Basically, estrogen is good for your hair, and testosterone is bad.

This is in part why women don't suffer androgenetic alopecia to the same degree as men: We have higher levels of aromatase action, particularly in the frontal hairline, which often preserves the very front line of hair, and hair loss is seen directly behind it.

Prolactin

It's also thought that high prolactin levels can contribute to hair loss, as this can increase DHEA levels. Because prolactin levels can be high in PCOS, if you have hair loss, it's worthwhile to have this checked.

Acne

Acne is a very troublesome skin condition related to the excess androgens found in PCOS. As we know, androgens are one of the most common causes of acne, and when androgens are high, acne can often be moderate to severe.

In the sebaceous gland of the skin, 5-alpha reductase converts testosterone into DHT. These androgens increase the formation of comedones in our skin by increasing sebum production from the sebaceous glands, causing abnormal changes in the skin cells. Bacteria accumulate, and papules and pustules then form on the skin. Studies have found that up to eighty-six percent of women with PCOS will have some degree of acne.[3] It's thought that the level of androgens and androgen receptors within the tissue of the skin are the greatest contributors to acne, rather than the overall level in the bloodstream. Younger women will tend to have more prevalent and severe acne. I often see that women with PCOS will tend to accumulate acne along their jawline or on the cheeks—the same areas you'll tend to see hirsutism—indicating an increase in androgen receptors in these areas in the skin.

Women with PCOS will often have early-onset acne, as the adrenal glands can activate earlier. Acne can also start later on, in a woman's twenties, thirties, or even forties. This is because androgens remain high throughout her lifespan. In fact, I've found that for many women who have significant acne that persists beyond the teen years, PCOS is likely hiding in the background. In addition, the acne of women with PCOS often doesn't respond to conventional acne treatments. This is because their acne is hormonal in origin. Even some of the stronger treatments for acne, such as isotretinoin, may work temporarily. However, due to hormonal imbalances, the acne can recur later.

Similar to acne, another skin condition is common in PCOS: hidradenitis suppuritiva. This involves small inflamed and often painful lumps under the skin that contain pus. Hidradenitis suppuritiva is most often found where skin rubs together in the armpits, groin, or under the breasts.

Treatments for Androgen Excess

A variety of treatments exist for androgen excess. These range from cosmetic treatments to pharmacological ones, including hormonally active natural treatments (such as spearmint tea and anti-androgenic herbs) to the most commonly prescribed medications (such as spironolactone) as well as various methods of hair removal. Of course, working on the root causes of androgen excess, such as inflammation, stress, and insulin resistance, will always be of great importance.

Conventional Medicine for Androgen Excess

There are several pharmaceutical treatments used to manage androgen excess. A review of them follows. There are also effective natural treatments with fewer side effects, which will be detailed next.

The Pill

Birth control pills are often the first-line treatment for the management of androgen excess in conventional medicine. The pill is composed of synthetic estrogens and progestins that suppress ovulation. When the week of inactive pills is taken each month, hormone levels drop abruptly, causing the lining to shed in a bleed, which looks similar to a period. The pill is typically used to override androgen excess symptoms and to stimulate monthly bleeding; however, it does nothing to support normal ovulatory cycles, as the ovary-pituitary axis is completely suppressed by its hormones.

The estrogen in birth control pills appears to have a beneficial effect on androgen excess symptoms, such as acne, hirsutism, and alopecia; however, the progestins in these pills can be androgenic and make matters worse. Unfortunately, high estrogen pills are not worth the risk, as they carry serious risks of breast cancer and blood clots.

When it comes to acne, most women know that it worsens when hormones fluctuate. Flares of acne often happen prior to ovulation, when testosterone rises, and after ovulation, when hormones levels change again. This is why for many women, non-cycled birth control pills that do not fluctuate in dosage produce the fewest breakouts.

The types of birth control pills that have the strongest androgenic properties and tend to aggravate acne, alopecia, and hirsutism are the ones containing levonorgestrel, norgestrel, etonogestrel, and DMPA. Medium-level androgenic pills include those containing desogestrel, gestodene, and norethindrone. Lower-androgen pills include norgestimate and cyproterone acetate. Anti-androgen birth control pills include drospirenone, which is closely related to the anti-androgen drug spironolactone.

Unfortunately, the types of pills that block androgens and tend to be the most effective also have the most risks for serious blood clots.

Drospirenone has been found to put women at increased risk of hypertension, blood clots, liver function disturbances, and even diabetes when compared to other progestins. In 2012, the FDA released an updated safety announcement explaining that pills containing drospirenone are linked to a higher blood clot risk than other birth control pills. In fact, two studies in the British Medical Journal found that there may be a two- to three-fold increased risk of deep vein thrombosis and pulmonary embolism in women taking these pills. Anti-androgen birth control pills can also contain more active and fewer inactive pills within a pack than other pills, resulting in an increased total amount of hormones taken. Although the anti-androgenic pills are the most risky when it comes to cardiovascular disease, all of birth control pills come with the risk of blood clots.

A recent study found that just three months of birth control pill use caused insulin resistance in women, and this effect was markedly worse in women with PCOS than those without the condition.[4] Also, it seems that birth control pills are not very effective for hirsutism in particular, as more than half of women end up with a poor response to this treatment.

Spironolactone

Spironolactone is the most popular anti-androgen therapy used for the treatment of hirsutism. It is also used to treat high blood pressure, as it is a diuretic that increases the amount of potassium in the body. This drug works in a few different ways: It blocks the androgen receptor and decreases testosterone production. It is strictly contraindicated in women who are trying to conceive. It comes with a long list of potential side effects, including causing irregular ovulation and periods. Of note, it can take more than six months to see benefit from using spironolactone for hirsutism, as it appears that the hair follicle remains altered for six months to a year even after androgen levels are normalized. Spironolactone doesn't help to reduce 5-alpha reductase activity, either. One of the main risks of this drug is elevated blood potassium levels, which can be serious. Other side effects associated with spirono-lactone include drowsiness and dizziness, low blood pressure, stomach upset, and headaches.

Finasteride

Finasteride is a drug that was developed to treat enlargement of the prostate in men. It works by inhibiting 5-alpha reductase, which can also be effective for hirsutism and alopecia. For women who may become pregnant, it is a very risky drug, how-ever, because it can cause abnormal development of the genitalia in male fetuses in the first trimester. Therefore, it is rarely given to women of reproductive age.

Flutamide

This is a newer drug that is anti-androgenic and has been effective for both hirsutism and acne. That being said, it has caused fatal hepatitis and is very expensive.

Steroids

Steroid therapy may be used for women with adrenal androgen excesses, such as high DHEA-S. The main steroids used are dexamethasone or prednisone. These sup-press the stimulation of the adrenal glands and reduce androgens. The negative of steroids is that they can cause weight gain even at low doses, so they are not well tolerated by many. In women with PCOS, this can be exceptionally problematic, as weight gain can definitely exacerbate the condition overall.

Natural Treatments for Androgen Excess

Before proceeding with natural treatments for androgen excess, try to determine if you have an excess of adrenal derived androgens (DHEA-S), ovarian androgens (testosterone), or a combination of the two. If there is an excess of adrenal andro-gens, the previous chapter on balancing your adrenals can show you how to reduce these androgens through stress reduction and minimizing stimulation of the adrenal gland by stress responses.

Of course, when you work on inflammation and insulin resistance, these will also help to decrease the output of androgens. Even with working on the underlying factors, androgen excess is stressful and often needs to be addressed directly, par-ticularly if there are bothersome symptoms, or if ovulatory problems still remain after addressing the aforementioned issues first. The following natural anti-andro-gen therapies can be effective for hirsutism and acne as well as androgenetic alope-cia and can be used by women with any form of androgen excess from adrenal or ovarian origin.

Licorice

Glycerrhiza glabra (also known as licorice), in a 2004 study titled "Licorice Reduces Serum Testosterone in Healthy Women," was found to significantly decrease testosterone levels in women after one month of treatment. The study concluded that licorice may exert its anti-androgenic action by blocking key enzymes involved in the production of testosterone. The steroids glycyrrhizin and glycyrrhetic acid have significant anti-androgen effects,[5,6] which may be helpful in reducing hirsutism, acne, and androgenetic alopecia in women with PCOS. Of note: Licorice can raise blood pressure and should not be used by those who have elevated blood pressure.

White Peony

Paeonia lactiflora (white peony) is another popular anti-androgenic herb. In tradiotional Chinese medicine, it is often combined with licorice in a ratio of 1:1 for the treatment of PCOS. Studies have found that this combination can decrease the production of testosterone without altering the production of androstenedione and estradiol.[7] I use this combination quite often in my practice for women with PCOS and find it to be helpful in the regulation of the menstrual cycle and for the reduction of androgenic signs. Peony and licorice formula is typically taken at a dosage of 2 grams 3 times per day, and up to 4 grams 3 times per day.

Green Tea

For women with androgenetic hair loss, hirsutism, or acne, *Camellia sinensis* (green tea) may be of benefit. The epigallocatechins (the most well-researched is EGCG) in green tea are 5-alpha reductase inhibitors, which decrease the production of dihydrotestosterone.[8] Dihydrotestosterone, as we know, is a major culprit in the skin conditions related to androgen excess. Green tea can also increase the sex hormone-binding globulin— the protein that binds up testosterone and prevents it from attaching to the receptors of the cells. This can be helpful for patients with elevated free testosterone.[9] Typical doses of EGCG— the active component of green tea— range from 400 mg to 600 mg per day in divided doses. Green tea also has a modest effect on fat burning. Drinking green tea is beneficial. One cup of green tea contains 50 mg of EGCG.

Reishi Mushroom

Ganoderma lucidum (reishi mushroom) has many health benefits. However, it also exerts a significant anti-androgenic action.[10] Research suggests that it can inhibit both Type 1 and Type 2 5-alpha reductase,[11] which can benefit the skin of women with PCOS. In addition, it appears to suppress the growth of cells that are stimulated by testosterone, suggesting that it may have a role to play as an androgen receptor blocker as well.

Typical doses of *Ganoderma* range from 1 to 5 grams per day, or it can be used in smaller doses as an herb in a formula. If you have an autoimmune condition, such as lupus, Hashimoto's thyroiditis, or rheumatoid arthritis, it may be best to avoid *Ganoderma,* as it is considered to be an immune-boosting herb.

Spearmint Tea

Spearmint tea at a dosage of one cup twice per day has been shown in two studies to have anti-androgenic properties.[12] Over a thirty-day period, spearmint tea brought about a significant reduction in free and total testosterone levels in a group of forty-two women with confirmed PCOS and hirsutism.[13]

Saw Palmetto

Serenoa repens (saw palmetto) is a well-known plant-derived anti-androgen. Saw palmetto is a 5-alpha reductase inhibitor of moderate strength that also shows promise for the treatment of androgenetic alopecia.[14] I use it often in formulas for acne as well as hirsutism. Typical doses of saw palmetto range from 150 to 300 mg daily.

Rosemary

As a topical therapy for androgenetic alopecia, *Rosemarinus officinalis* (rosemary) leaf extract was found in a 2013 study to improve hair regrowth in mice with androgen-induced hair growth interruption. Rosemary leaf extract showed inhibitor activity upward of 82.4 percent in inhibiting 5-alpha reductase. It also decreased the binding of DHT to androgen receptors.[15] I recommend rosemary to all of my patients suffering from alopecia and find that results of new hair regrowth are seen within six to eight months.

Typically, three to four drops of rosemary oil are applied with a carrier oil, such as jojoba, and then applied gently to the scalp for thirty minutes prior to washing the hair. It is also recommended not to wash the hair more than three times per week, if at all possible.

Melatonin

Melatonin is a therapy that has been found to increase the anagen hair rate for women with androgenetic alopecia. It works best for occipital and frontal hair loss. One study used melatonin topically in a 0.1 percent solution, which resulted in significant improvement in alopecia.[16] As we discussed earlier, hair loss is often related to oxidative stress. It's likely that the antioxidant properties of melatonin were at play in protecting the hair follicles from destruction.

Phytoestrogenic Plants

As we know, estrogen is an anti-androgen. In women with PCOS, there is a strong imbalance in the ratio of estrogen to testosterone, with the androgens dominating. Estrogens can help to calm down the skin, reduce hirsutism, and improve hair growth. There is a category of plants that have properties that can counter the effects of elevated androgens. Phytoestrogens may help some patients with acne and aggravate others, as any flux of hormones can be aggravating to acne. As such, the following treatments may be best utilized for those with alopecia or hirsutism.

Soy

I do not usually recommend soy for women with PCOS. The reason is that the vast majority of soy is genetically modified and has unknown effects on our future health. Although soy does contain a wide range of isoflavones, I generally will choose other plants with the same properties that are organically produced.

Kudzu Root

Kudzu root (*Pueraria*) is a plant that contains a significant amount of isoflavones, including puerarin, daidzein, daidzin, and genistein. These are mild compounds that fit into the slot of the estrogen receptor, yet have a very weak effect. However, they can help signal the cell's internal mechanisms, helping the cell to respond to hormonal cues. Kudzu root as a phytoestrogen, however, may aggravate acne in some individuals, so it is recommended more for patients with alopecia and/or hirsutism rather than those with acne. Typical doses of Kudzu root range from 1 to 3 grams per day in divided doses.

Black Cohosh

Cimicifuga Racemosa, or black cohosh, is categorized as a phytoestrogen, though there is now conflicting information suggesting that this may not be the case. That being said, as outlined in Appendix A, it does appear to have benefits for women with PCOS and can improve LH/FSH ratios and increase ovulation rates. Recent research has also found that it can reduce the proliferation of prostate cancer cells, an androgen-dependent tumor. However, the study also found that it could reduce the prostate cancer regardless of its androgen receptor status.[17] In addition, Black Cohosh has been found to inhibit 5-alpha reductase, indicating that it may have benefits for skin that exhibits symptoms of excessive testosterone in women with PCOS.[18]

Iron—A Special Consideration for Hair Loss

It's crucial to consider your iron levels with androgenetic alopecia in the mix. Research has found that optimal levels of stored iron (known as ferritin) must be maintained to keep the hair in an anagen (growth) phase for the longest period of time possible.

A 2002 study found that of women with increased hair shedding and decreased hair volume, ninety-five percent had a serum ferritin of less than seventy.[19] Another study found that treating iron deficiency, bringing the average ferritin levels from thirty-three to eighty-nine, caused a significant decrease in hairs entering into the shedding phase. A ferritin level of under forty has also been linked to a significant increase in telogen hairs. The hair follicles contain stores of ferritin that encourage them to grow.

Ferritin is produced from the iron we take in through our food by the liver. As a woman's ferritin drops, the liver stops producing more ferritin from iron. Instead, it must be used to produce hemoglobin in the developing red blood cells within the bone marrow. Ferritin is then taken from the tissues, including the hair follicles. Without enough ferritin, the hairs that were previously growing will go into the telogen (falling out) stage. Typically, once a hair has entered the telogen phase, it will fall out within two to four months. As a result, it's always important to remember that hair loss was likely caused by an incident that happened between two to four months prior.[20]

I often recommend a ferritin goal of eighty for women with androgenetic alopecia. In fact, I would state that addressing iron levels in the body is the single most important factor for women with hair loss. Once iron levels are built up, the hair will no longer enter the telogen phase as often, and hair loss will gradually improve. This is a slow process given the time it takes to grow new hair and the fact that many hairs may have already entered the telogen phase from when iron levels were low and, as such, are pre-programmed to fall out. Typical needs for iron are 8 mg per day. However, in deficiency, much larger doses from 35 mg and upward may be needed to build up iron stores.

There are several well-absorbed and generally well-tolerated forms of iron, including heme iron (one hundred percent absorption), iron bisglycinate (twenty percent absorption), iron citrate (eighteen percent absorption), and carbonyl iron (one hundred percent absorption). For those with severe gastrointestinal side effects from even the irons listed here, most patients say that both heme and carbonyl iron produce the least constipation and stomach upset. This is because their high absorption rate allows less to be consumed.

Another hormonal consideration women with PCOS should know about when it comes to hair loss is the thyroid, which is often a culprit. Low thyroid levels can decrease the production of sex hormone-binding globulin (SHBG), which normally binds up all of that troublesome testosterone. Therefore, low levels of SHBG allow testosterone to act more freely and will only make your hair fall out more. Insulin resistance also decreases SHBG. So dealing with our central insulin resistance is *always* the key for any androgenic symptom.

Topical Treatments for Acne

In conventional medicine, topical treatments like benzoyl peroxide, topical antibiotics, and topical vitamin A preparations like retinoic acid may provide various results. Again, since the condition is hormonal, their effect may be limited. Yet, at the same time, topical treatments can help women while working on fully balancing their hormones.

Fortunately, there are several effective natural topical treatments for acne, which are sometimes a necessary part of treatment, as they can help manage sebum accumulation and bacteria. With acne, working both from inside out and outside in results in the best outcome.

Salicylic Acid

Salicylic acid (SA) is technically a natural product, although it has been isolated and made into a variety of commercial products that you see on drugstore shelves. Made from white willow bark, it has been clinically proven to reduce acne outbreaks by unclogging pores and removing dead skin cells to prevent further congestion and pimple formation.

Tea Tree Oil

Tea tree oil is a natural product that can reduce the number of lesions in women with mild to moderate acne. It's antimicrobial and anti-inflammatory. Typically, tea tree oil is applied twice per day and seems to provide improvement in just six weeks. One study comparing it to topical antibiotics (erythromycin) found that it was significantly better at reducing outbreaks.[21] When compared to benzoyl peroxide at five percent, tea tree oil was comparable in its ability to reduce acne lesions.[22]

Japanese Cypress Oil

This extract has proven anti-acne action. A very recent study compared tea tree oil to lactobacillus-fermented cypress essential oil.[23] It found that both treatments were effective; however, the cypress oil came out on top, reducing lesions by 65 percent and 52.6 percent for inflammatory and noninflammatory lesions, compared to tea tree oil at 38.2 and 23.7 percent. Sebum extraction was decreased by thirty percent after eight weeks in the cypress (LCFO) group. A variety of other essential oils have been studied for acne, including rosemary and lavender.

Glycolic or Alpha Hydroxy Acid

These are natural acid products that can be helpful for the treatment of acne. For mild cases, these natural products can help to kill acne bacteria and also to reduce comedones that are the precursors to acne. Another benefit of glycolic/alpha hydroxy acids are that they give the skin a glowing appearance, removing dead skin cells from the surface. It can be applied daily at a concentration ranging from five to ten percent. Typically it's best to start at a lower concentration—glycolic acid can create a burning or tingling sensation as well as peeling—as you work up in concentration. Occasionally, glycolic acid can also be applied as a stronger peel, which has also been shown to significantly reduce acne bacteria.

Cosmetic Treatments for Hirsutism

Since hair follicles often accumulate over time, many women will need to employ a variety of hair removal methods. These should be used along with natural treatments to reduce androgens.

Plucking and Waxing

Plucking and waxing are commonly used treatments for hirsutism. However, they are generally not optimal, because women with PCOS are much more prone to developing acne and folliculitis. Once plucking occurs, the follicle can become inflamed and clogged. This can even result in pigmentation or scarring. However, for some women, waxing and plucking are well tolerated, and in these cases may be an excellent solution.

Shaving

Shaving generally works quite well for hirsutism. The negatives are, that it must be performed daily in many cases, and it can be stressful psychologically. Regrowth is often quickly visible, and for women who have significant hirsutism, this can be stressful.

Electrolysis

Electrolysis is an excellent method of hair removal. It is permanent and generally can be effective. In rare cases, it can cause scarring. The other negatives are that it is time consuming, expensive, and can be painful.

Laser

Laser is one of the most popular approaches for hirsutism. It is permanent and scarring is rare. The negatives are that it is expensive, and it works best on women who have light skin and dark hair. For women with darker-toned skin and darker hair, it is generally less effective, and the same goes for women with blonde hair and light skin. In short, laser works best when there is a pigment contrast.

Overall, androgen excess is a central issue for women with PCOS, stalling ovulation and blocking healthy cycles, changing hair growth, and triggering acne. It also causes many women to feel that they have lost their femininity, since signs of androgen excess are visible and often difficult to manage. I hope that this chapter has provided you some solutions to these distressing concerns. Anti-androgen treatments always work best with good management of insulin resistance, inflammation, and stress—the underlying triggers of androgen excess in PCOS..

Chapter 6

STEP 5. ADDRESS HORMONAL IMBALANCES

I feel safe in the rhythm and flow of ever-changing life.
—LOUISE HAY

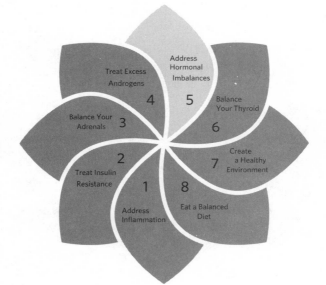

Madeline was a twenty-six-year-old woman who had experienced abnormal menstrual cycles throughout her entire life. Her menstrual cycles would make an appearance once or twice per year, and when they did, they were exceptionally heavy and painful. Madeline often had to call in sick to work for the first days of her period, spending the day in agony with a heating pad pressed up against her belly. Madeline was diagnosed with PCOS early on as a teenager and was placed on birth control pills rather promptly. At the age of twenty-five, she had read about the risks associated with hormonal birth control and decided to come off of the pill for good.

Unfortunately, this did not turn out so well. Her periods didn't return with a normal, regular cycle, as she had so optimistically hoped. Just as they were before, her cycles arrived few and far between, and there were no signs of ovulation on her test kits. Madeline came to see me at the clinic to get some help and to effectively regulate her hormones. We started with some testing to look at the function of her pituitary gland and how it was communicating with her ovaries, and therein lay the issue. We began a course of herbal medicine along with natural progesterone cream. Just as we had hoped, her cycles returned in two months. With more work on nutrition and addressing stress, over eight more months, Madeline was able to achieve regular twenty-nine-day ovulatory cycles without the help of any medication for the very first time in her life.

The Hormones in the Menstrual Cycle

As women, we are synonymous with change. Our fundamental nature shifts throughout our lives, and our hormones change their complex patterns in a similar style. This is the result of a variety of feedback mechanisms, ebbing and flowing, creating what we experience as our monthly cycles.

There are three main areas in the body to know about when it comes to understanding our female hormones. The first two of these are located in our brains. The hypothalamus is the hormone control center of the brain. It's located deep within our brains, and one of its most important functions is to link our nervous system to our hormonal system. The hypothalamus communicates with a small gland that is directly in front of it, the pituitary. You've probably heard of the pituitary gland already, as it's really the master gland, controlling the various hormonal systems in the body.

The hypothalamus, being a very sensitive area of the brain, picks up on a lot that is going on around us and directs the pituitary to adjust the hormonal environment in the body. The pituitary then, under direction of the hypothalamus, sends out messages to the ovaries, the thyroid, the adrenal glands, and more.

Since this book is about PCOS, we will be placing a lot of emphasis on the ovary. The ovary is our main estrogen- and progesterone-producing gland, and it is responsible for overall female hormonal balance and the process of ovulation itself.

The ovary picks up on the signals from the pituitary gland and responds by growing follicles for each ovarian cycle. These follicles, which house the eggs, are responsible for producing the vast majority of female hormones found in the body. The hypothalamus, pituitary gland, and ovaries are three key areas that work in concert, talking to each other though complex feedback loops and adjusting as needed.

The Ovary and the Follicles

One of the most important things to understand is that when we ovulate, our eggs do not just pop up out of nowhere. They grow very slowly for around three hundred and sixty days from tiny primordial follicles before they are developed enough for ovulation. When we are newborn babies, we already have the tiny follicles containing the eggs that we will ovulate throughout our lives.

The follicles reside in dormancy for many years, waiting patiently for their turn to be ovulated. As we reach puberty, some of these eggs, housed snugly within their follicles, will begin their preparation for ovulation. During this yearlong process, known as folliculogenesis, the cells of the follicles that surround the egg will grow and multiply.

As the follicle develops, its many cells multiply and begin producing hormones. There are two parts to the follicle's structure: the inner part, known as the granulosa, and the outer part, known as the theca. The egg is sheltered deep within the follicle, at the center of the granulosa cells.

As the follicle develops in preparation for ovulation, the granulosa produces estrogen, and the theca produces testosterone. Several eggs develop together for a given cycle, the best one of the batch is selected for ovulation, and the rest will undergo a process of disintegration. In fact, the vast majority of all follicles that undergo folliculogenesis will not make the journey. As the chosen follicle for any given cycle approaches ovulation, it produces increasing amounts of hormones, namely estrogen, along with some testosterone.

The pituitary gland plays an important role in this process. When it senses that there is a low level of estrogen, as is the case when the menstrual period begins each cycle, it responds by sending hormonal signals to the ovary to prepare an egg for ovulation. The hormone used to prepare the follicles for ovulation is known as follicle-stimulating hormone (FSH).

The pituitary uses FSH to stimulate the ovary and then selects the strongest, best follicle to survive. The other follicles will disintegrate. As the selected follicle gets bigger, its granulosa cells produce estrogen. This peak of estrogen is a signal to the pituitary gland that a follicle is mature and ready for ovulation.

The pituitary gland responds to the high level of estrogen by sending out a pulse of luteinizing hormone (LH). This pulse of LH is what ovulation test kits pick up. LH is produced in a short, powerful surge, triggering the egg's final development and release by causing the follicle to rupture.

After ovulation, the now-empty follicle's work is not yet done. The follicle undergoes a massive transformation, turning into an important structure called the corpus luteum. The corpus luteum has a crucial role to play, as it is the key producer of progesterone in women. The corpus luteum is needed for hormone balance and for implantation of the embryo, should an egg be fertilized.

The corpus luteum should last around fourteen days before it disintegrates. During its lifespan, it performs the important task of releasing progesterone along with some estrogen. The corpus luteum is an independent preprogrammed structure. It requires a huge amount of blood flow and energy to keep itself alive. The corpus luteum doesn't get any feedback from the pituitary like the ovary does, and when it has reached its lifespan of two weeks, it simply breaks down.

Knowing that the corpus luteum is formed out of the cells of the follicle, its ability to produce sufficient progesterone is totally dependent on the quality of the follicle that has developed for many months before. The cells of the follicle that become the corpus luteum must be structured well enough to survive and produce hormones through to the very end of the luteal phase.

At the end of this fourteen-day period, the corpus luteum breaks down and progesterone and estrogen levels drop, causing the shedding of the endometrial lining through the menstrual period. The pituitary gland senses low levels of estrogen and responds by releasing FSH again, preparing the ovary to develop another group of follicles for the next cycle.

How the HPO Axis Is Disturbed in PCOS

As you can see, there is a lot of back and forth communication between the hypothalamus, the pituitary gland, and the ovaries in a woman's menstrual cycle. For women with PCOS, we know that this communication is quite disrupted.

In women who do not ovulate, there is a hormonal flatline. When it comes to the hypothalamus in PCOS, it is thought that there are primary changes in the way it sends signals to the pituitary gland. The hypothalamus tells the pituitary gland what to do by sending out pulses of a hormone called gonadotropin-releasing hormone (GnRH). When it pulses slowly, it triggers the release of FSH. When it pulses more quickly, it triggers the release of LH. As mentioned previously, teenage girls tend to have faster pulses of GnRH, causing a predominance of LH, but this gradually shifts to its typical female pattern of slow pulsing at the beginning of each cycle. The elevated progesterone and estrogen levels in the luteal phase typically slow down the pulses of GnRH in preparation for the next cycle. This is not so in PCOS.

In women with PCOS, the GnRH pulses do not slow down enough in response to estrogen and progesterone levels, and as a result, GnRH continues pulsing too fast. The predominance of fast pulsing results in overproduction of LH across the cycle. LH causes the ovary to make more testosterone, which inhibits ovulation (as shown in Figure 6-1).

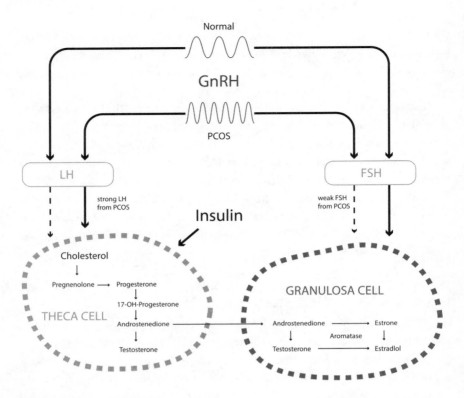

Figure 6-1: Hypothalamus Pituitary Ovary

In PCOS, the follicles have an unusual structure: The outer theca layer is too thick when compared to the inner granulosa layer. This is caused by too much insulin and LH—common problems in PCOS.

As mentioned before, the theca cells are responsible for producing testosterone, and the follicles begin to oversecrete testosterone relative to estrogen. Too much testosterone within the ovary slows down follicular development. There is no mid-cycle surge of estrogen as the follicles grow, and there is no responding surge of LH to trigger ovulation.

As you can see, this is a vicious cycle that flattens our natural hormonal rhythms. The all-important hormonal feedback loops that keep ovulation going are completely lost.

Over time, follicles may partially develop in a PCOS ovary as they attempt to grow. As this happens, estrogen begins to rise, but testosterone overrides it, and the follicle comes to a premature halt. Estrogen doesn't get the opportunity to rise high enough to stimulate a surge in LH and a successful ovulation.

Even if ovulation is achieved, the quality of the follicle in PCOS is usually decreased. The corpus luteum, the progesterone-producing structure of the follicle, is often not as robust and may disintegrate early. As a result, even when they do ovulate, many women with PCOS have a serious deficiency of progesterone.

A Special Hormone to Consider: AMH

Another more recently discovered hormone, known as anti-Mullerian hormone (AMH), also comes into play. Women with PCOS have too many of what are known as antral follicles. These antral follicles include the stalled follicles just described, and they secrete plenty of AMH.

This hormone is often tested in fertility clinics to assess the number of eggs in a woman's ovary. As would be expected, the number is often highest in young women and lower as women get older. However, for women with PCOS, AMH levels are often elevated due to both the increased number of follicles in the ovary and the fact that the follicles themselves produce increased amounts of AMH in PCOS.[1] As such, AMH is a useful test for ovarian hormone imbalance for women with PCOS. Table 6-1 shows the normal ranges of AMH. If you are above this range for your age, this is a marker of PCOS. An overabundance of AMH slows down follicle development, further perpetuating the cycle of hormonal imbalance and anovulation.

New information also suggests that AMH plays an important role in the brain as well as in the ovary. High levels of AMH can excite neurons in the hypothalamus, causing them to release GnRH at a higher frequency.[2] This causes the pituitary to make more LH, adding back into the cycle of androgen production in PCOS.

Table 6-1: Typical Age-Related Ranges for AMH

AGE		
Under 33 years old	2.1–6.8 ng/dl	15.0–48 pmol/L
33–37 years old	1.7–3.5 ng/dl	12.14–32.13 pmol/L
38–40 years old	1.1–3.0 ng/dl	7.8 –21.42 pmol/L
41+ years old	0.5–2.5 ng/dl	3.57–17.85 pmol/L

These are compiled from evidence and our own clinical experience at the clinic working with fertility patients and women with PCOS. (McCulloch 2015; Yoo et al. 2011; Gleicher 2016)

Lab Testing for Female Hormones and Ovarian Function

Women with PCOS often benefit from the following tests to assess hormones and ovarian function. If you have menstrual cycles and are ovulatory, you should have the tests completed on the days indicated. If you do not, these can also be done on any random day. Day 1 of a menstrual cycle is the first morning you wake up with a full flow of menstrual bleeding (not including spotting).

Table 6-2: Tests to Assess Hormones and Ovarian Function

HORMONE	NOTES
FSH, LH	Should be done on Day 3 of your cycle.
	Reference: Both FSH and LH are typically between 4-8 miU/mL on Cycle Day 3.
	In most cases, FSH is higher than LH on Cycle Day 3, although sometimes the two numbers can be equal.
	In women with PCOS, the LH is often higher than FSH and can be double or even triple the FSH level.
Estradiol	Should be completed on Day 3 of your cycle. Reference: 25-75 pg/ml or 91-275 pmol/L
Progesterone	If possible, seven days after ovulation is the ideal time to test progesterone.
	Reference > 18 ng/ml or 57 nmol/L confirms that ovulation has likely occurred.
Prolactin	This can be tested on any cycle day. This is a pituitary hormone that inhibits ovulation and can be increased in PCOS.
AMH	This can be tested on any cycle day. Please refer to previous table for reference ranges.

(Mayo Medical Laboratories 2016; Woo et al. 2015; Buyalos, Daneshmand, and Brzechffa 1997)

Conventional Therapies

Synthetic Hormones

Once again, the most commonly prescribed conventional therapy for women with PCOS is the oral contraceptive pill. This involves the use of synthetic hormones, which completely override the entire hormonal system. Using birth control pills will, in fact, lead to a period every month, but they will not help you to ovulate. The synthetic forms of progesterone found in the birth control pill are particularly risky. They've been linked to blood clots and strokes. As mentioned in chapter 5, the birth control pills most commonly used for PCOS are the ones that have the highest risks, and women with PCOS are already at increased risk for blood clots.

One issue that is common in women with PCOS is something called post-pill amenorrhea, which is the lapse of the menstrual cycle and ovulation for quite some time after women have stopped taking birth control pills. The reason that I believe women with PCOS are more prone to this is that the hypothalamic-pituitary-ovary connection doesn't have the same ability to kick back into its feedback loops after a hormonal change. I've seen women with PCOS take upward of eighteen months for their periods to return after stopping the pill. That being said, not all women experience this. It just seems to be more common in PCOS when compared to the general population.

Progesterone Withdrawal Therapy

Another commonly used intervention is the administration of a dose of progesterone, often for seven days, to induce a menstrual bleed. This, once again, does not induce ovulation. However, this is something I do not consider as harmful, particularly if a woman has not had a period in months. It is likely necessary to induce shedding of the lining after three to four months without menstruation (particularly if a woman commonly has very long intervals between her periods) to prevent a condition called endometrial hyperplasia.[3] Endometrial hyperplasia is an overgrowth of the endometrial lining due to a deficiency of progesterone and prolonged exposure to estrogen. Over time, this can increase risk for endometrial cancer. There are natural forms of progesterone, such as bio-identical progesterone creams, that can also be used to induce a period.

Natural Therapies for Female Hormone Regulation

The rebalancing of the hormonal axis in PCOS is something that depends on many factors. This is why I address it after what I consider to be blockages, such as insulin resistance, stress, androgen excess, and inflammation. That being said, there are some effective natural therapies that can help to reset the hormonal axis. My favorite approach when it comes to natural therapies is to use herbal medicines. These gently stimulate changes in hormones, which can provide feedback to the hypothalamus, pituitary, and ovary. These treatments should not be used long term, but rather for a treatment course to reinstate hormonal feedback loops.

In women who do not have regular menses, I will often create a cycle for them, numbering days as we go. In women with PCOS who do have a cycle, we always count Day 1 as the first day a woman wakes up with a full menstrual bleed. The following are some of my favorite herbal combinations for women with PCOS.

White Peony and Licorice

White peony root and licorice can help reinstate cycles for women with PCOS—particularly for those where androgen excess is overriding the ovulatory process. This formula, which is comprised of a one to one ratio of each plant, can be used all cycle long and can improve ovulation rates. A study on thirty-four Japanese women with PCOS found that 7.5 grams of this formula per day was able to improve the FSH to LH ratio, reduce testosterone levels, and improve the ratio of estradiol to testosterone.[4]

Black Cohosh

Black cohosh is helpful in many ways for women with PCOS. It has been found to improve the FSH to LH ratio, increase progesterone levels, and induce ovulation. It may be used during either phase of the cycle. However, it should not be used by anyone with liver disease, and liver enzymes should be monitored to ensure that you can tolerate this herb.

Black cohosh has also been found to modulate the pituitary, reducing the secretion of LH.[5] For women who are taking clomiphene, the most common first-line fertility drug, research has found that black cohosh can improve the negative effects of the drug on endometrial lining and cervical mucus and improve luteal phase progesterone and pregnancy rates.[6, 7]

Vitex

Vitex, or chaste tree, is exceptionally effective for women who have elevated prolactin.[8] It is clear that it reduces prolactin through effects on the dopaminergic system of the brain.

In initial studies and older herbal textbooks, vitex was reported to increase LH, stimulating ovulation and progesterone production. Of course, this created great confusion as to how this herb actually worked, when clinically it does seem to benefit many women with PCOS who have inherently high LH levels. It has, in traditional herbal medicine, been used a cycle regulator, so something within its action on the hormonal system wasn't quite fully explained by this older research.

Fascinating newer research has determined that much of the way vitex works lies within its action on the brain. Its ability to regulate the cycle involves its action on the brain's dopaminergic and opioid systems. Effects on the pituitary hormones are secondary. With respect to LH, clearly of concern for women with PCOS, further studies have found differing results than preliminary findings indicated. As an example, in a recent study on male mice, vitex was found to reduce the levels of LH.[9]

In yet another study on female mice, it was found to have no effect on LH in repro-
ductive-age animals, yet was able to lower the hormone in menopausal rats.[10] Con-
fused yet? Don't be. I'm going to explain how vitex can and does affect the pituitary
hormones but does so at a higher regulatory level within the brain.

The main thing to understand with vitex is that it clearly does not increase or
decrease specific hormones in the same way that taking a hormonal drug would, or
this would be very evident from the numerous recent studies on this plant.

What it does appear to do is to act on the brain, regulating hormones from a
higher level. Clinically, in certain situations, when a woman has low LH levels, for
example, you may see the LH rise up in preparation for ovulation when she is taking
the herb. However, in other situations, such as menopause or PCOS, where LH is
high, you may see it reduce. And in other situations, it may have no effect at all.

New research suggests that vitex likely binds to different types of opioid receptors that are found within in the brain.[11] According to one study, vitex affects natural
beta opioid levels, with an increase of 105 percent after just five days of treatment.[12]

The opioidergic system is very important, as it controls certain actions of the
reproductive system. It inhibits the hypothalamic-pituitary-adrenal axis, reducing the negative impact of this axis on GnRH, LH, and FSH.[13] In other words, it
stops your brain from triggering the production of stress hormones. And the most
important action it has with respect to female hormones, and especially to women
with PCOS, is that opioids slow down pulsing of the hypothalamic master hormone
GnRH.[14]

Now, let's think back to the problem with GnRH that is present in women with
PCOS. GnRH pulses too fast. The role of progesterone after ovulation is to slow that
pulsing. When the pulse slows down, the pituitary starts making FSH to grow an
egg and shifts away from making LH. Women with PCOS don't have enough progesterone to slow the pulsing down. In addition, they appear to have hypothalamic
resistance to progesterone.

Recent studies have found that women with PCOS have clear dysfunction of
the opioid system of the brain.[15] This is the exact system that vitex works on. Insulin resistance in PCOS further aggravates dysfunction of the opioid system. So in
women who are insulin resistant, the opioid system's function may be significantly
improved by working on that factor first.

Overall, vitex helps regulate the hypothalamus by slowing down its rapid pulsing
and allowing FSH to take predominance. FSH is what allows a follicle to grow and
produce estrogen, causing a surge of LH that triggers ovulation. So when we think
now about what vitex does, and about how LH and FSH work, it isn't as simple as
raising one hormone or another. Vitex can help get the concert of hormones back in
order, so they can start to self-regulate once again.

We now know that vitex can work on the dopaminergic system of the brain and reduce prolactin levels (which, if high, inhibit ovulation). We also know that it works on the opioidergic system, slowing GnRH pulses and reducing LH. When used in the right way, vitex can be exceptionally beneficial for women with PCOS. So again, you can tell if you are stuck in a state of fast GnRH pulsing by testing your LH, which will be high much of the time.

Vitex's opioidergic effect is likely part of why numerous studies demonstrate its efficacy in reducing the mood-related symptoms of PMS and improving painful periods. I believe this system may be one of the reasons that women with PCOS are more prone to depression, anxiety, and other mood disorders. There are different ways of using vitex, but I would like to show you the two main ways that I use it in my practice.

The first is when a woman has moderately high LH and is ovulating, but ovulation is delayed (for example, women who have a thirty-two to forty-five-day cycle), I use vitex only in the luteal phase. I prescribe it in the morning as a single dose. The reason for this is that prolactin follows a diurnal circadian rhythm—with highest levels during the night when it is dark. On rising, prolactin should drop. Women who have high prolactin often have difficulty with this circadian rhythm and can be best assisted by reducing prolactin in the morning, following the natural circadian rhythm.

The reason I use vitex only in the luteal phase is to encourage the slowing of the GnRH pulse and to reduce LH and increase FSH to prepare for the next cycle. I find that once the slow pulsation is established at the start of the cycle, the pituitary will respond well to the subsequent rise in estrogen. I find that this often takes several cycles to have full effect. Typically four to six months on vitex will help to establish good regularity.

The second way I use vitex in my practice is for women who have longer periods of time between cycles or who have complete amenorrhea. I prescribe it for them daily. In these women, GnRH pulsing is fast on a continuous basis. Therefore, vitex can be beneficial when used in a continuous manner to break what can sometimes be a stubborn hormonal pattern.

The method of dosing is the same. It is taken in the morning. Once semi-regular ovulation is established and ovulation can be detected, I then switch over to the first method. Once regular cycles have occurred for three cycles, I will stop the herb.

I typically dose vitex at 1,500 mg in the morning (typically a 6:1 or 5:1 extract). Both tinctures and dried extracts can be effective. Choose them carefully, however, as many commercial products do not have enough of the flavonoid components to effect the mu-opioid system, including apigenin, luteolin, isokaempferide and cas-ticin. The diterpenoid components of vitex work to reduce prolactin through the dopaminergic system, so these are important as well. It is unfortunate that there are many inferior herbal products on the market.

Peony and Cinnamon

These herbs are another powerful combination for women with PCOS. Typically, they are used throughout a woman's entire cycle and are often helpful for those with slower metabolic function and insulin resistance. Together, these two herbs have been found to reduce testosterone, reduce LH, improve the LH/FSH ratio, increase ovulation rates, increase the granulosa's production of estradiol, and increase luteal phase progesterone. Dosing typically ranges from 6 to 10 grams per day in divided doses.

Dong Quai

Angelica root (*Angelica sinensis*), or dong quai, is an herb with a long tradition in traditional Chinese medicine. It is a hormonal regulator and is a phytoestrogen that can bind to estrogen receptors and weakly activate them. This can be beneficial for women with PCOS who are deficient in this key female hormone. It has been shown to activate estrogen responsive genes within the reproductive organs, turning on mechanisms that may have lain dormant. For women with PCOS, I have found it to be an excellent herb, particularly when used in the follicular phase of the cycle. In addition to this, dong quai has been found to increase the generation of red blood cells in a process known as hematopoiesis. As such, for women who have very light periods, or iron deficiencies in addition to PCOS, it may be an ideal hormone-regulating herb. Dong quai is often dosed at 200 to 500 mg, three times daily.

Full-Cycle Formulas

Peony and licorice work well for lack of cyclicity with androgen excess predominance, whereas peony and cinnamon are used for lack of cyclicity with insulin resistance predominance and poor circulation. Both combinations can be used for the duration of your cycle.

Cycle Day Formulas

For women who have predominant hypothalamic pituitary dysfunction, I have often used variations on the following based on time of the cycle. This is a more advanced herbal prescription and often requires the support of an herbalist or a naturopath. There are innumerable other variations that can be used depending on your needs. However, this would be best assessed by a practitioner who can devote adequate time to your entire case.

Follicular Phase Formula

The following can be used during the follicular phase:

- *Angelica sinensis* (fifty percent)
- *Paeonia lactiflora* (thirty percent)
- *Cimicifuga racemosa* (twenty percent)

Luteal Phase Formula

The following can be used during the luteal phase:

- *Vitex agnus-castus* (eighty percent)
- *Glycerrhiza glabra* (twenty percent)

In my clinic, I prescribe tinctures and will customize the amounts and vary the formulas. You can purchase quality tinctures from reputable local herbalists or through your local naturopathic doctor. You can have the tinctures compounded for you, or you can mix them yourself at home.

The dosage for these tinctures is one teaspoon in the morning and one in the evening. Typically, many herbs are made in a 1:4 extract (meaning one part herb with four parts solution). If your extract differs concentration-wise, please adjust your dosage accordingly. For example, if you have purchased a 1:2 extract, you should reduce your dose by approximately half.

Chapter 7

STEP 6. BALANCE YOUR THYROID

Every mile is two in winter.

—GEORGE HERBERT

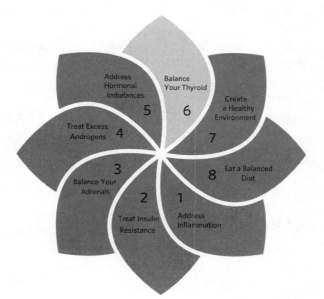

Alyson was a thirty-two-year-old woman with PCOS. Throughout her life, she had dealt with having highly irregular menstrual cycles and hirsutism. Like many women with PCOS, she had difficulty losing weight and found that no matter how many different types of diets she tried, she just couldn't shed the pounds. Alyson only got around two periods per year, and her doctor had prescribed medroxyprogesterone to induce periods every so often. Fortunately, Alyson was able to achieve pregnancy naturally, but after she had the baby, she just didn't feel well.

Her doctor thought she might have postpartum depression, as she was very depressed and felt extremely tired. Her libido was nonexistent, and as thrilled as she was to have a brand-new, beautiful baby, she just didn't have the energy to make it through the day. In fact, on some days, Alyson could barely get out of bed. Alyson was also extremely constipated. Sometimes, there would be days between visits to the bathroom for her. She couldn't lose her baby weight like her friends did. She was frustrated, sad, and exhausted. She wondered if this was another terrible side effect of PCOS?

After a medical checkup, it was discovered that Alyson had a fairly significant thyroid disorder. Her thyroid stimulating hormone (TSH) level was very high at 8.4. The doctor told Alyson that this was most likely the source of her extreme fatigue, depression, constipation, and difficulty losing weight. Alyson wondered how she could have such bad luck to have both PCOS and hypothyroidism?

Well, in fact, the two conditions *are* related. Women with PCOS are more at risk for the negative effects of hypothyroidism, and the two conditions work together to create a vicious cycle of exhaustion, weight gain, insulin resistance, hormonal imbalance, and many more unpleasant symptoms. Let's learn more about the thyroid and how important its optimal function is to women who have PCOS. This section will contain a lot of scientific information, so hang on tight and get ready to learn!

Thyroid Disease: What Is It?

If you have read about thyroid disorders in the past, you'll know how very common they are. Around ten million Americans are thought to suffer from hypothyroidism. Risks for hypothyroidism include a past family history of any type of autoimmune disease, a family history of thyroid disease, past exposure to radiation on the neck or upper body, or having been pregnant within the past six months (as happened in Alyson's case).

The most common cause for hypothyroidism in the developed world is an autoimmune disease called Hashimoto's thyroiditis, where the immune system attacks the thyroid gland, rendering it underactive. Other causes include environmental ones, such as radiation exposure, iodine deficiency, and mercury and bromide (a chemical found in pesticides and plastics) exposure.

Women with PCOS should definitely have their thyroids carefully investigated, as the symptoms of hypothyroidism can aggravate PCOS. There is also an increased risk of autoimmune thyroid disease in women with PCOS.

Symptoms of Hypothyroidism

It's important to be able to recognize hypothyroidism. The symptoms of hypothyroidism can range from mild to intense and life altering. They can start suddenly at any time; however, the chance of developing thyroid disease increases with age. And as in the case of Alyson, the risk sharply increases in the postpartum period or after any hormonal shift such as in the menopausal transition. Some of the symptoms include—

- Fatigue
- Feeling cold
- Hair loss
- Weight gain
- Difficulty losing weight despite changes in diet and exercise
- Dry skin
- Constipation
- Muscle cramps and aches
- Depression
- Irritability
- Poor memory and concentration
- Changes in menstrual cyclicity
- Low libido
- Increased risk for miscarriage and infertility

You might think that many of these symptoms look very similar to the symptoms of PCOS. As we know, women with PCOS are already at risk for infertility and early pregnancy loss. Many find it difficult to lose weight through diet and exercise, and they suffer from fatigue, depression, and anxiety. As you can see, there's a significant overlap of symptoms between PCOS and thyroid disease, despite the fact that they are two very different conditions. As these conditions can certainly exacerbate each other, it's very important to ensure that the thyroid is functioning optimally in women with PCOS.

We will now go a bit deeper into why thyroid hypofunction is so problematic in women with PCOS.

Hypothyroidism and Insulin Resistance

Research suggests that low thyroid function can aggravate the insulin resistance in PCOS.[1] So, if you need to have your hormones assessed, it's helpful to understand the thyroid hormones and how they work. Let's go through a brief review of the different thyroid hormones and their functions (see Figure 7-1). The following are the hormones that may be tested for by your doctor.

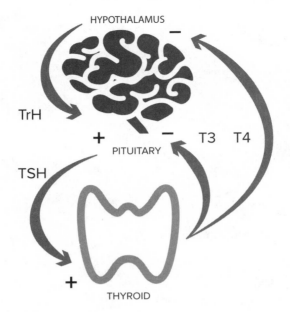

Figure 7-1: Thyroid Function

Thyroid Lab Testing
- TSH
- Free T3
- Free T4
- Reverse T3
- Anti-thyroid peroxidase antibody
- Anti-thyroglobulin antibody

Thyroid-Stimulating Hormone

Thyroid-stimulating hormone (TSH) is the hormone that is secreted by the pituitary gland, the pea-sized hormonal "master gland" located in the brain. When the brain, specifically the hypothalamus and pituitary gland, perceives that there is a low level of thyroid hormone in the body, the pituitary gland responds by increasing the secretion of TSH.

TSH then travels to the thyroid gland, which responds by releasing thyroid hormone. When thyroid hormones are in abundance, the pituitary reduces its output of TSH to keep levels from rising too high.

As such, most patients who have hypothyroidism have increased TSH levels. When thyroid function is low, the pituitary gland tries to compensate, pushing the thyroid to make the needed hormones.

In the world of testing, TSH is definitely the most popular lab marker ordered by most physicians for the assessment of the thyroid. Many doctors believe it is the only test required to assess thyroid function. I disagree with this, as do many other naturopathic doctors, functional medicine practitioners, and thyroid specialists. I have found that optimal thyroid function depends on the full concert of thyroid hormones. In some cases, thyroid hormones themselves may be low, yet the TSH can be within normal range, which results from specific systemic conditions. In addition, the optimal ranges for TSH are controversial, with hot debate occurring in the medical community. Please see the section that follows for a discussion on optimal TSH levels for women with PCOS.

TSH

- Released from the pituitary gland
- Stimulates the thyroid to make T4 and T3
- Normal range between 0.4 and 3.0 miU/mL
- Optimal range between 1.0 and 2.0 miU/mL

Thyroxine

Thyroxine (T4) is one of the two primary thyroid hormones released by the thyroid gland. The thyroid hormones' main function is to stimulate the metabolism of the cells and tissues in the body. T4 is made by attaching four iodine molecules to the amino acid tyrosine, with the help of a special protein known as thyroglogulin. Thyroxine is the least powerful of the two thyroid hormones, but it is also the most abundant and has the longest half-life. T4 is actually considered to act more as a prohormone, rather than a hormone. It is a reservoir that can be converted into the more active T3 as needed. The thyroid gland secretes around 100 mcg of T4 every day. As far as testing, free T4 is ordered more often than total T4.

Triiodothyronine

Triiodothyronine (T3) is the most powerful thyroid hormone and is made of three iodine molecules attached to the amino acid tyrosine. It has a powerful effect on all metabolic processes in the body. T3 is considered to be three to four times more potent than T4. The ratio of T4 to T3 is 20:1, and T4 is converted to T3 as needed by the body if conversion processes are functioning optimally. T4 is converted to T3 by special selenium-containing enzymes called deiodinases (as shown in Figure 7-2). The thyroid gland secretes approximately 6 mcg of T3 every day. An additional 24 mcg of T3 is produced by the conversion of T4 into T3 in the tissues of the body. As far as testing, free T3 is ordered more often than total T3.

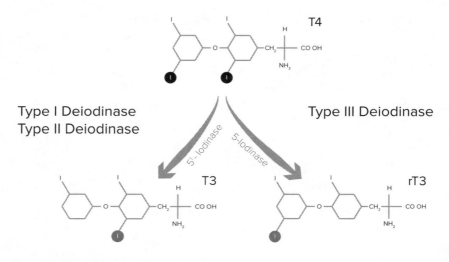

Figure 7-2: Thyroid Hormone Conversion

Deiodinase Enzymes

These important enzymes work to convert the T4 that is in reservoir into T3. There are several different types of deiodinase enzymes. Type 1 deiodinase is found mainly in the liver and the kidneys. Type 2 deiodinase is found in the brain in cells known as astrocytes, and Type 3 deiodinase is found in the neurons of the brain. As you can see, the body has complex mechanisms for controlling its metabolic rate, which differ from organ system to organ system. In some cases, the deiodinase enzymes may be downregulated. This reduces the conversion of T4 into T3, causing less-active thyroid hormones to be available to the body. This causes symptoms of hypothyroidism, despite the fact that the TSH and T4 levels may be within "normal" ranges.

Free Thyroid Hormones vs. Total Thyroid Hormones

There are carrier proteins in the blood that bind up thyroid hormones so they cannot act on the cells. At any given time, most of the thyroid hormones are actually bound up. As such, it is considered to be more relevant to test the "free" hormones, which are the hormones available to act on the tissues of the body. The free hormones are able to directly activate the cells in the body and often correlate closely to a patient's signs and symptoms of hypothyroidism.

Free T4

- Thyroid hormone produced by the thyroid gland
- Mostly inactive
- The most abundant unbound thyroid hormone
- Not bound to carrier proteins

Free T4

This is a measure of the amount of unbound thyroxine hormone. Only a very small fraction of T4 hormone is free and active. Again, free T4 is mostly a storage hormone that can be converted to T3 as needed by the body.

Free T3

This is the unbound T3 that can act on the cells. Free T3 is a very metabolically active hormone and is quite powerful. Many patients say they feel best when their free T3 levels are within a certain range. It's important to note that thyroid hormones are quite variable from hour to hour. As such, it's important to test thyroid hormones at a consistent time of day (often in the morning), and to repeat testing if the numbers appear to be abnormal. Despite its importance, free T3 is not routinely ordered. Most patients have to request this test.

Free T3

- Most metabolically active thyroid hormone
- Converted from T4 as needed by the body
- Not bound to carrier proteins

Autoimmune Thyroid Testing

Anti-Thyroid Peroxidase Antibodies
Anti-thyroid peroxidase (anti-TPO) antibodies attack an important enzyme involved in thyroid hormone production known as thyroid peroxidase. Thyroid peroxidase assists in the release of iodine, so it can be used to form T4. Antibodies against thyroid peroxidase can block the ability of the thyroid to produce thyroid hormone. Anti-TPO is the most common thyroid antibody, occurring in ninety percent of patients with Hashimoto's thyroiditis and seventy-five percent of those with Grave's disease, two of the most common types of autoimmune thyroid disease. As these thyroid antibodies act within the thyroid gland itself, they can cause thyroid cell damage by activating immune processes within the gland.

Thyroglobulin Antibodies
Anti-thyroglobulin (Tg) antibodies are specific for thyroglobulin, which is a protein that is involved in thyroid hormone production. They are found in seventy percent of patients with Hashimoto's thyroiditis and thirty percent of patients with Graves' disease. Around thirty percent of patients who are positive for anti-TPO will also be positive for anti-Tg.

Reverse T3

- Mostly inactive
- Third most abundant thyroid hormone
- Used to turn down the metabolism by the tissues in times of stress or illness
- Optimal ranges: 0–25 ng/dl
- Ratio of free T3 to reverse T3 should be twenty or more
- Reverse T3 reference range 0–25 ng/dL

Reverse T3

Reverse T3 is an isomer of T3, meaning it has a very similar structure, with a positional difference of where one of the iodine molecules is placed. Reverse T3 is the third most common thyroid hormone made by the thyroid gland. However, it is rarely tested.

Most of the reverse T3 is made outside of the thyroid gland by the cells of the body. Reverse T3 is metabolically inactive and can be used by the body to "turn down" the metabolism when needed. In situations of stress or illness, T4 is converted into reverse T3 instead of T3 through a particular deiodinase enzyme known as 5-deiodinase (as seen in Figure 7-2). In these situations, reduced activity of deiodinase enzymes in the tissues of the body and decreased liver uptake of reverse T3 results in higher levels of reverse T3.

Interestingly, reverse T3 is inert and does not have any of the metabolic effects of T3. Because it is structurally similar, it can enter the cells and bind to the thyroid hormone receptors just as the strong metabolic stimulator T3 would. As such, high levels of reverse T3 can block some of the metabolic processes by competing with the receptors in the cells. In fact, part of reverse T3's function is to preserve energy in times of starvation, illness, or high stress. Cortisol in excess can increase reverse T3 for this very reason.

The pituitary gland is quite sensitive to T4 and rapidly switches off its production of TSH when T4 levels rise. As such, in cases where free T4 is normal, yet free T3 is low and reverse T3 is high, TSH may also appear to be normal on testing. This is the exact reason testing *TSH is not enough to assess thyroid function in a woman with PCOS who may have high cortisol, high insulin, or other factors that increase the production of reverse T3.* When having your thyroid checked, it is best to request the full panel.

Typically, the ratio of free T3 to reverse T3 should be good. In other words, you want to have much more of the active T3 when compared to the inactive T3. Even if your reverse T3 is within the recommended range, if the free T3 is low in comparison, this indicates that your body is trying to shut down its metabolism. There is a handy calculator to determine your free T3 to reverse T3 ratio at: http://www.stopthethyroidmadness.com/rt3-ratio/. If your ratio is below twenty and you have the symptoms of hypothyroidism, then it is likely you have a problem with reverse T3.

Low T3 Syndrome or Low Conversion

In times of metabolic stress or disease, T3 levels decrease. This condition is known as euthyroid sick syndrome, or low T3 syndrome, and occurs when TSH is quite normal, yet T3 is low and reverse T3 is high. Adding to this effect, the lower levels of T3 slow down metabolism so the body doesn't eliminate reverse T3, and it further accumulates in the blood. In less severe cases, you may see that the T4 is much higher within the reference range than T3 is. For example, many patients have a free T3 at the bottom of the range of values, indicating that conversion may be poor.

It's important to note that TSH doesn't correlate to your metabolism. Both TSH and serum T4 do not correlate well with thyroid hormone levels within the cells of our bodies. As mentioned earlier, the conversion of T4 to T3 is decreased in situations of physiologic stress (this can include emotional stress or even physical stressors, such as lack of sleep or starvation diets).

Free T3 is the most accurate marker of thyroid function in situations of physiological stress. As such, in women with PCOS who are dealing with less than optimal physical balance, free T3 is a key hormone to test.

The transporter for reverse T3 is also affected by stress on the body. Without good transporter function, reverse T3 can't get into the cells, and it remains in the blood.

As such, reverse T3 is a good marker for reduced cellular T4 and T3 levels not detected by TSH. When the reverse T3 is high, we know that external physiological stresses are decreasing your metabolic function and may be causing symptoms of hypothyroidism in your case.

A Case of Normal TSH and High Reverse T3

One of my patients, Diana, had many of the symptoms of hypothyroidism in addition to the PCOS that many of the female members in her family suffered from. She was diagnosed with hypothyroidism several years before and had been placed on levothyroxine. As a result, her TSH had reached the "normal" range and her symptoms had improved.

But within the past year, she began to feel symptoms creeping back. Diana was feeling cold and tired. She had gained twenty pounds that she couldn't shake and just didn't have the motivation to do the things in life that she enjoyed. Diana, a college professor who taught literature, was quite good at research and had certainly done a good amount of investigating into her own case.

She went to her doctor, certain that she would need an increase in thyroid hormone dosage. However, her TSH labwork came back in the optimal range, with a level at 1.75. Diana then requested to have her free T3, free T4, and reverse T3 tested. Her ratio of free T3 to reverse T3 was at eight, which was exceptionally low.

After coming to see me in the clinic, we reviewed her entire case history and found that Diana had been experiencing extreme stress at her job in the last year, as well as very heavy periods. We performed some bloodwork, taking a look at her iron stores (ferritin), which came back low at eight, and her adrenal glands through a salivary cortisol test, which revealed adrenal fatigue. Knowing that these two factors could increase conversion to reverse T3, we began to supplement Diana's diet with a high quality iron supplement, a B complex vitamin, and various supplements to support her adrenal health.

Diana placed more emphasis on sleep, yoga, and meditation. We also added some supplements to increase conversion into T3, which we will discuss at the end of this chapter. By the time four months had passed, Diana felt like new again: She felt warm and was back to her old energy levels. She also lost ten pounds through the same program she had followed consistently to keep her PCOS under control. Best of all, Diana's free T3 to reverse T3 ratio increased to twenty-two!

Insulin and Thyroid Hormones

Numerous studies have found that diabetes, insulin resistance, and metabolic syndrome reduce the conversion of T4 to T3 and promote the formation of reverse T3. As such, women with PCOS who commonly have insulin resistance often have higher than average reverse T3 levels. As overall thyroid hormone levels, including reverse T3, are highly variable, it may be useful to conduct repeated testing to get an average of your levels.

High insulin levels also increase the activity of one of the key enzymes involved in thyroid hormone production, deiodinase-2. Yet, instead of turning T3 into active thyroid hormone, insulin resistance causes much of it to turn into the inactive reverse T3.

The pituitary gland is smart. It can detect increases in deiodinase activity and respond by making less TSH (as shown in Figure 7-1). If only TSH is tested, this can give the false impression that everything is fine. This is why we can't use TSH alone as a reliable marker of tissue thyroid levels for women with insulin-resistant PCOS.

Subclinical Hypothyroidism and PCOS

Studies show that women with PCOS have higher TSH levels and are also more likely to have subclinical hypothyroidism when compared to age-matched controls without PCOS.[2] This may be in part due to some of the effects related to insulin resistance.

First, it may be important to discuss the difference between subclinical hypothyroidism and what is known as overt hypothyroidism. In overt hypothyroidism, a patient will have an elevated TSH, and one or both of T4 and T3 are low. In subclinical hypothyroidism, patients will have an elevated TSH while T4 and T3 are in the normal range.

When it comes to defining subclinical hypothyroidism, there is great controversy. Several studies have suggested a lower cutoff than the conventional 4–5 miU/L to define subclinical hypothyroidism. The National Academy of Clinical Biochemistry's (NACB) laboratory guidelines state that greater than ninety-five percent of rigorously screened normal euthyroid (meaning normal thyroid function) volunteers have serum TSH values between 0.4 and 2.5 mIU/L.[3]

Other sources, and most in the conventional medical profession, suggest using the typical cutoff of 4–5 miU/L. That being said, it appears that women with PCOS may have a different optimal range than others, as the impacts of insulin resistance do affect the thyroid function.

There is little research on the use of free T3 (fT3) and free T4 (fT4) tests themselves for the diagnosis of subclinical hypothyroidism, but countless patients, naturopaths, and doctors who practice nutrition and natural medicine have noticed that being toward the upper end of the range seems to correlate with patient symptom improvement.

In my own naturopathic practice, I find it generally best to treat the patient first and look at the lab values as only a guideline, as patients feel best at different personal ranges for thyroid markers. Imagine a world where we treat the patient and their symptoms first.

Some evidence does suggest that women with PCOS do better with a tighter range for TSH. As stated earlier, TSH production is lower in the presence of insulin resistance, which can make a poorly functioning thyroid look normal on testing. The thyroid hormones themselves may still not function optimally. Within the cells, conversion can decrease, and the amount of reverse T3 can accumulate. We already know the hazards and unpleasantries of having high reverse T3. In women with PCOS, metabolism should be at the most optimal level possible, since there are enough hurdles to jump over already with respect to hormones.

TSH Levels and PCOS

Although TSH is not the best overall marker to assess thyroid function, there is some research studying this particular hormone in women with PCOS. A 2009 study looked at a group of 337 women with PCOS. All of the women were assessed for the key markers of PCOS, including hirsutism, acne, and menstrual irregularity.[4]

What the researchers found was that the women who had the lowest levels of insulin resistance also had the lowest TSH values (under 2 miU/L). Women with the highest TSH values tended to have the most severe insulin resistance. Interestingly, this was not related to weight: Subclinical hypothyroidism caused insulin resistance in women in all weight categories. This provides further evidence that insulin resistance hinders thyroid function.

The study concluded that a TSH above 2 miU/L was associated with insulin resistance in PCOS. Another study following women with PCOS found that those who had a TSH greater than or equal to 2.5 mIU/L had a higher body mass index, higher fasting insulin levels, higher total testosterone, and lower sex hormone-binding globulin concentrations in comparison with women with a TSH under 2.5 mIU/L.[5]

Having low thyroid function aggravates all of the symptoms of PCOS. Thyroid function is associated with our metabolism of glucose. So just as insulin resistance can disrupt thyroid function, the reverse is also true. A woman with PCOS who has simultaneous hypothyroidism is entering into a vicious circle of hormonal dysfunction. In women with PCOS, there is a markedly increased risk for cardiovascular disease, and this same risk is found in hypothyroidism.

When thyroid dysfunction is added to PCOS, the chances of metabolic, hormonal, and cardiovascular risks increase dramatically. For women with PCOS, we want thyroid function to be optimal, not just to be on the borderline of acceptable. An optimal TSH range for a woman with PCOS may be between 1 and 2.5 mIU/L.

Again, the existing research on this topic is focused on TSH, but it is also highly likely that an optimal range exists for fT3 and fT4 in PCOS. In my practice, I have found that values at the top one-third to one-fourth of the range are often most beneficial for symptom relief and metabolic health in women with PCOS.

Sex Hormone-Binding Globulin, the Thyroid, and PCOS

Changes in thyroid function can also influence levels of a protein known as sex hormone-binding globulin (SHBG). SHBG sticks to androgens that float around in the blood, rendering them unable to activate the cells.

When SHBG levels are low, androgens can run rampant in the body, causing the unpleasant androgenic symptoms of PCOS. Typically, high levels of insulin push down SHBG and, as a result, can be used as a marker for overall insulin levels. The lower the SHBG, the higher the insulin will often be.

Thyroid hormones generally increase the levels of SHBG,[6] and in patients who have hypothyroidism, there is often a deficiency of SHBG. When added to the preexisting deficiency in PCOS caused by insulin resistance, androgenic symptoms, such as hair loss, acne, and hirsutism, can be far worse when thyroid function is low.

Ovarian Volume and Cysts in Hypothyroidism

Hypothyroidism can look much like PCOS on an ultrasound all on its own. Hypothyroidism increases the size of, and promotes, cyst formation within the ovaries. Hypothyroidism also causes collagen and compounds known as mucopolysaccharides to deposit within various organs of the body. When deposited in the ovaries, these deposits can affect hormone synthesis and inhibit healthy ovulation, which is not something women with PCOS need. That being said, this type of cyst is *not* the same as the "cysts" in PCOS.

Hypothyroidism

- Increases ovary size
- Promotes cyst formation
- Interferes with ovulation

A 2011 study compared two groups of women with hypothyroidism—one group with polycystic ovaries and the other with normal ovaries—to a group of women with normal thyroid function. The researchers discovered that the hypothyroid women had larger ovaries overall. Providing thyroid hormone replacement therapy reduced the size of the ovaries in both groups of hypothyroid women and improved TSH, fT3 and fT4, prolactin, estradiol, free testosterone, and total testosterone levels.[7]

Surprisingly, for all of the hypothyroid women in this study, the polycystic ovaries completely disappeared when thyroid function was restored, although that doesn't mean their PCOS was cured. Although many of the women experienced more regular periods on thyroid hormone replacement therapy, half of the women with polycystic ovaries still did not begin to cycle regularly.

As you can see, hypothyroidism can cause a condition that in some ways looks similar to PCOS, but they are certainly not the same condition. If thyroid replacement hormone completely reverses PCOS, then it's not actually PCOS. However, many women with PCOS also have hypothyroidism, so it is important to investigate it, since it can make matters much worse. This is why I consider hypothyroidism an important factor in the treatment of PCOS, even though it is not actually a part of the polycystic ovary syndrome diagnostic criteria.

Autoimmune Thyroiditis and PCOS

There is a strong relationship between autoimmunity and PCOS. Autoimmunity occurs when the immune system turns against tissues of the body. The most common type of autoimmune disease is Hashimoto's thyroiditis. Hashimoto's is the leading cause of hypothyroidism in women of reproductive age. Numerous studies have found that there is a very clear correlation between Hashimoto's thyroiditis and PCOS.

A 2012 study found that women with PCOS had a 65 percent increase in thyroid peroxidase antibodies (a marker for Hashimoto's thyroiditis) and a 26.6 percent increase in the incidence of goiter, when compared to age-matched subjects.[8]

An analysis conducted in 2013 found that in a total of six studies involving 1,605 women, there was an increased prevalence of autoimmune thyroiditis, increased serum TSH, increased anti-TPO antibodies, and anti-Tg antibodies in women with PCOS when compared to control groups.[9]

A recent study showed that women suffering from PCOS-related infertility who also had high anti-thyroid antibody levels were also significantly more likely to be resistant to clomiphene. The study went on to conclude that autoimmune thyroid disease is associated with poor treatment response in infertile women who suffer from PCOS.[10]

Thyroid-Related Risks Increased in PCOS

- Anti-TPO antibodies
- Anti-Tg antibodies
- Poor conversion of T4 to T3
- Higher TSH levels
- Goiter

PCOS Symptoms Magnified by Thyroid Conditions

- Insulin Resistance
- Increased cholesterol and lipids
- Slow metabolism and weight gain
- Infertility
- Irregular ovulation
- Risk of miscarriage
- Clomiphene resistance
- Mood disorder
- Hair loss

At this point, one thing is absolutely clear: All women with PCOS should have their thyroids evaluated thoroughly with the tests outlined earlier in the chapter.

Some patients with PCOS require thyroid hormone replacement therapies, but there are also PCOS patients with mild thyroid hypofunction or Hashimoto's who benefit greatly from therapies such as adrenal support, thyroid specific nutritional supplements, and dietary changes, to reduce autoimmunity.

Metabolism, Leptin, and Thyroid Hormones

Leptin, discovered in 1994, is an important hormone that is part of the hunger system, which we discussed in chapter 3. To briefly review, leptin is made by the fat cells in our bodies. It turns off feelings of hunger and increases feelings of satisfaction. When leptin levels are low, we get hungry and food becomes more rewarding.

As we learned in the chapter on insulin resistance, the more fatty tissue that a person has, the more leptin they will produce. After a while, the brain becomes "leptin resistant" and can no longer respond normally to leptin. The reward system doesn't cue a person to stop eating when leptin is high, and overeating can easily lead to obesity. It's a vicious cycle, and it explains a lot about why it can be so challenging for people to lose weight.

So how does this relate to the thyroid? We all know that dieting and low calorie intake slows down the metabolism. Food restriction and weight loss cause the thyroid gland to makes less T4 and T3, which lowers the overall metabolic rate.[11] It appears that, at least in part, resistance to leptin may be associated with this decrease in thyroid hormones. In a body that is leptin resistant, yo-yo dieting and other extreme methods of food restriction can be extremely problematic.

The Pituitary Gland, Leptin, and the Reverse T3 Connection

In women with a higher body mass index, complex interactions between thyroid hormones, leptin, and the hypothalamic-pituitary axis are altered. In a study investigating the connection between the pituitary gland, leptin, and the thyroid, a group of rats were fed a high-calorie diet that caused insulin resistance, leptin resistance, and weight gain. Researchers found a thirty-five percent decrease in the deiodinase activity in the pituitary gland for rats on the high calorie diet. As we just learned, deiodinase is responsible for the conversion of T4 into T3. As would be expected, these animals had 1.5 times the amount of reverse T3 as the animals fed the standard diet![12]

Leptin resistance increases reverse T3, effectively slowing down our thyroid hormone's ability to activate our metabolisms. All of this causes a cascade of events, which affects the body's natural hunger mechanism and even the thyroid function, all of which slow down our metabolism further, creating a vicious cycle.

The same study also concluded that it's likely that leptin works at the level of hypothalamus, the part of the brain that is involved in regulating our thyroid. In PCOS, the brain itself can become leptin resistant, reducing thyroid function despite excess energy stored in fat cells that is available to be burned.

Treatments for Hypothyroidism and Hashimoto's Thyroiditis

Fortunately, thyroid conditions are usually very treatable. Depending on the severity and cause of thyroid dysfunction, treatments ranging from vitamins and minerals to thyroid replacement hormones may be needed.

Pharmaceutical Treatments

Following are the pharmaceutical options for those requiring thyroid hormone replacement.

Levothyroxine

This is a synthetic thyroid hormone that is chemically identical to the T4 that is secreted by your thyroid. This is a prescription drug, and it is the most common medication prescribed for hypothyroidism. Dosages often start at 25 micrograms and move upward. Side effects of levothyroxine include tremors, headache, nausea, vomiting, diarrhea, nervousness, irritability, excessive sweating, changes in menstrual cycling, and temporary hair loss. It is important to note that each patient may require different dosages to reach a state of normal thyroid function. As T4 is mostly a storage reservoir, the use of levothyroxine requires the patient's body to convert T4 into T3. Levothyroxine contains lactose, so if you have an intolerance, you may want to choose another product.

Dessicated Thyroid

Natural thyroid hormones, made from the thyroid glands of pigs and powdered for therapeutic use, are often prescribed by functional medicine doctors. These products were developed over a century ago and are still used today. They contain a combination of both forms of thyroid hormone, T4, and T3, in a ratio of 4:1, and thus the patient is not required to convert as much T4 to T3. Each patient's response tends to be unique, with some patients feeling best symptomatically on levothyroxine and others feeling better on dessicated products. Before embarking on any thyroid hormone replacement therapy, it is important to consult with a specialist who has experience in the prescription of these products. Dosages begin at 0.25 grains of dessicated thyroid.

T3 products

This is the most potent form of thyroid hormone, chemically nearly identical to T3. It acts on the body to potently increase the metabolic rate and increases the body's sensitivity to chemicals such as adrenaline. It has a faster onset of action and a shorter half-life than T4 preparations. Some doctors will use this in addition to T4 therapeutically; however, it is not a commonly used medication, and typically only very specialized doctors will prescribe it.

Natural Treatments

A variety of vitamins and minerals are essential for healthy thyroid function, and natural anti-inflammatory approaches can be used to help calm autoimmunity.

Iodine

Iodine is one of the most important nutrients for thyroid function. Iodine deficiency, which used to be restricted to parts of the world where iodine was depleted in the local soil, has more recently been affecting developed nations like the US and Canada. It is estimated that more than eight hundred million people are deficient in iodine worldwide, and this may be related in part to industrialized nations getting a large part of their food supply from nonlocal sources. Foods rich in iodine include seafood, milk, and eggs. Overall, vegans are more at risk for iodine deficiency. Food sources of iodine may vary, depending on the mineral content of the soil and food supply.

Iodine deficiency in the developed world can also be caused by bromide intake. Bromide is an element found in pesticides, medications, and fire-retardant chemicals. Bromide competes with the same receptors that are used in the thyroid gland to hold iodine, blocking the ability of the thyroid to make thyroid hormones. Urine tests are available that can determine iodine levels in the body and whether or not bromides are displacing the uptake of iodine in the thyroid.

Iodine deficiency can cause major problems for women with PCOS. It can cause hypothyroidism, which can impact fertility. As such, it's really important to get enough. I often recommend a minimum of 250 mcg per day of iodine. Many prenatal vitamins do not have this amount.

Some clinicians use high doses of iodine to treat hypothyroidism. I do not recommend this unless you are under the supervision of an experienced physician. The use of high-dose iodine must be done with great caution and with the correct preparation beforehand. It must be balanced properly with selenium and other minerals to prevent aggravation or uncovering of latent thyroid autoimmunity. In some cases, however, iodine can be very helpful, and there are many patients who report improvements in their condition with this therapy. Typically, up to 1 mg of iodine is safe per day for most women to consume without risking any negative effects.

Table 7-1: Iodine Content of Foods

FOOD	IODINE (MCG) PER SERVING
Seaweed, 1 g	16-2984
Cod, baked, 3 ounces	99
Iodized salt, ¼ tsp	71
Shrimp, 3 ounces	35
Egg, 1 large	24
Banana, 1 medium	3
Turkey, light meat, 2.5 oz	30
Chicken, 2.5 oz	11-13
Beef, 2.5 oz	11-14
Green peas, 0.5 cup	3-4
Beans (pinto/kidney) 0.75 cup	19-28

Sources:

Dietitians of Canada - Food Sources of Iodine. http://www.dietitians.ca/Your-Health/Nutrition-A-Z/Minerals/Food-Sources-of-Iodine.aspx.

Office of Dietary Supplements - Iodine. https://ods.od.nih.gov/factsheets/Iodine-HealthProfessional/#h3.

Selenium

Selenium is one of the most important minerals needed for thyroid function. It's also common to be deficient in selenium, since the soil's content varies greatly from location to location. Selenium is used to convert T4 to T3 and benefits patients with autoimmune thyroid conditions. It regulates the production of harmful reactive oxygen species, which can damage thyroid cells. In patients with autoimmune thyroiditis, it can decrease anti-thyroid antibodies and improve the ultrasound structure of the thyroid gland. Typical doses for selenium range from 200 to 400 mcg per day. Brazil nuts, although an excellent source of selenium, tend not to be consistent in their content. For patients with autoimmune thyroid disease, I recommend supplementing selenium, particularly in the form of selenomethionine, since it is such a key nutrient.

Zinc

Zinc acts as an antioxidant within the thyroid, and deficiency of zinc has been associated with hypothyroidism. Zinc is used in the formation of TSH and to convert T4 into T3. As such, zinc been shown to increase free T3 concentrations. For patients with hypothyroidism, zinc is recommended at a dosage of around 15 to 30 mg per day. It's also important to consider that long-term supplementation with zinc can create an imbalance of copper in the body. As such, these two minerals are often given in combination: typically 1 mg of copper per 15 mg of zinc. Alkaline phosphatase levels in the serum can be low when zinc is deficient.

Ashwagandha

Ashwagandha, also known as Indian ginseng, is a helpful herb for hypothyroidism and also for adrenal health. There is some research suggesting that in some cases it may be an androgenic herb. The degree to which that occurs is still unknown, and I have seen many women with PCOS take ashwagandha without any negative effects. It may be helpful for women with PCOS who do not have extremely high androgen levels, in particular as an adjunct herb as part of a formula. Ashwagandha has been found to increase serum T4 and T3 in animal studies. More research will need to be done to determine the effect of ashwagandha on women with PCOS. Dosing for ashwagandha ranges from 300 to 1000 mg per day.

Gum Guggul

Although this plant extract has a funny name, it has a serious benefit for thyroid health. This relative of the myrrh gum tree has long been used medicinally. It's been shown to stimulate the thyroid in animal studies. And as an additional benefit for women with PCOS, it can reduce high cholesterol and improve metabolic function. Gum guggul contains compounds, known as ketosteroids, which can increase the uptake of iodine by the thyroid gland and improve the activity of the enzymes in the thyroid. It can improve the ratio of T3 to T4.[13] Typical dosages of gum guggul (also known as commiphora mukul) are 125 mg twice daily.

Blue Flag Iris

Iris versicolour, or blue flag iris, is a small wild botanical used in the 1800s to help with the lymphatic system. In modern times, we've learned that it's also a helpful anti-inflammatory agent and can reduce enlargement of the thyroid in patients who have Hashimoto's thyroiditis. A typical dosage of *Iris versicolour* is 750 mg per day.

Coleus Forskohlii

Coleus, a member of the mint family that grows on the mountainous terrain of India, Nepal, and Thailand, is a plant that can activate T3 and T4 secretion from the thyroid cells in an action that is quite similar to TSH. It improves iodide uptake from the thyroid gland and increases the production of thyroid hormones. It also increases something known as cyclic AMP, which can raise the metabolic function and lower blood sugar, both of which are beneficial for most women with PCOS. A typical dose of coleus is 50 mg per day.

For patients with a strong autoimmune condition, such as Graves' disease or Hashimoto's thyroiditis, I'd also recommend embarking on a gut-immune healing program, as outlined in chapter 9.

When it comes to thyroid conditions and PCOS, each patient is truly unique in her needs. Hormonal systems are complex and intertwined, and doctors should look at the specific relationships that exist in each and every patient to create a plan that helps to restore optimal metabolic and hormonal health.

Chapter 8

STEP 7. CREATE A HEALTHY ENVIRONMENT

We do not inherit the earth from our ancestors,
we borrow it from our children.

—NATIVE AMERICAN PROVERB

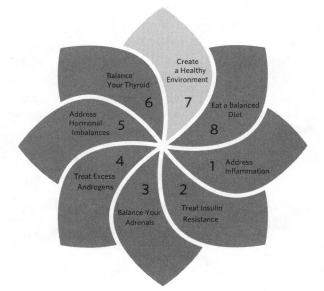

PCOS is a rapidly growing epidemic. The increased incidence of PCOS coincides with industrialization and the introduction of a wide variety of chemicals into our environment. Unfortunately, there is not much available data on the health effects of chronic low-dose exposure to many of these compounds, yet new ones are introduced every week. Most of these chemicals are known as either persistent or semi-persistent organic pollutants (POP), because they don't break down, accumulate in the food chain, and persist in our environment. POPs can have additive and synergistic effects, so it's quite difficult to truly understand the far-reaching consequences they have on human health. As many of these chemicals have hormone-like effects, there has been a good amount of investigation into their connection with PCOS. What has been found is more than concerning.

Epigenetics and Environmental Influencers on PCOS

We do know for certain that there are strong genetic factors involved in PCOS, with inheritance clearly seen within families. We also know that there are some blood markers, including adiponectin, which can predict those children who are at risk for developing PCOS later on. So we know that the condition is present prior to puberty. Although genes may be present in an individual's cells, there are times and factors that increase the activation of the genes. The activation of genes by environmental factors is known as epigenetics, and it's thought that this plays a major role in the evolution and transmission of PCOS through generations.

Hormonal Influences of Environmental Chemicals

Our environment has become a hostile place, particularly when it comes to hormonal development. Because certain industrial and agricultural chemicals disrupt the very way that our endocrine system functions, they are commonly known as endocrine-disrupting chemicals (EDC). Pregnant mothers, babies, and children are the ones most vulnerable to this. The processes that govern reproductive development are most active in these groups and can be permanently changed by the influence of EDCs.

EDCs can change how hormones are produced, the way that they attach to receptors, and the ways that they interact with each other. Hormones can accumulate in our tissues over a lifetime. They also accumulate in the environment. Over time, they become more and more pervasive. And as you'll see, their harmful effects compound with each generation, which is certainly cause for concern.

EDCs have been recognized as a major public health crisis, as they are clearly connected with many different human pathologies. PCOS is no different. In fact, environment may be one of the major important factors in its course and persistence.

BPA and Effects on PCOS

One of the most well-researched examples of an EDC is bisphenol A (BPA). BPA is a chemical commonly used in the production of plastics that has a particularly strong relationship to PCOS. BPA is a xenoestrogen, a chemical that imitates estrogen that can activate or block estrogen receptors in various tissues of the body, including the ovaries, uterus, and brain. Chemical xenoestrogens are serious environmental hazards that can disrupt hormonal function in both men and women and accumulate and persist in our fatty tissue for decades.

BPA has been widely used in infant bottles, water bottles, medical devices, cash register receipts, and as lacquers to coat food cans and water supply pipes. It is also used in dental composites and sealants. BPA can leach into our food from the resin coating of canned foods and from plastic products, such as water bottles. BPA has even been found in breast milk. The exposure to BPA is extremely widespread. The 2003–2004 National Health and Nutrition Examination Survey conducted for the Centers for Disease Control and Prevention (CDC) found detectable levels of BPA in ninety-three percent of urine samples from people aged six years and older. Pregnant women, infants, and children are most vulnerable to the effects of BPA. More than 150 peer-reviewed studies have found negative health effects from exposure to BPA. These effects include reduced fertility, changes in ovarian health and structure, breast and prostate cancer, and developmental problems in children.

PCOS is no different. Concerning research has been brought forth giving us insight into the power of this chemical on our hormonal systems. A 2015 study found that teenaged girls with PCOS had higher levels of BPA than girls without PCOS and that the amount of BPA in their systems correlated to the degree of their androgen excess.[1]

This was independent of obesity, indicating that BPA exposure is directly related to PCOS and its severity.

Another study found that BPA levels in women with PCOS correlate with fatty liver and markers of low-grade inflammation like C-reactive protein (CRP) and interleukin 6 (IL-6).[2]

BPA can bind to both estrogen and androgen receptors in our body, and it can affect the production of hormones as well as the development of the follicles within the ovary, known as folliculogenesis.

As you can imagine, BPA can also affect the very function and structure of the ovary. It stimulates the theca cells of the follicles, causing them to produce androgens, and it also interferes with the production of estrogen. In addition, BPA reduces the activity of enzymes that break down testosterone, resulting in the further accumulation of androgens. The high androgen levels in PCOS also reduce the liver's ability to clear BPA from the circulation, causing a vicious cycle of BPA accumulation, endocrine disruption, and androgen excess in the body.

To make matters even worse, BPA also affects our fatty tissue. It has been found to reduce the production of adiponectin from fat cells as well. Adiponectin is the protective anti-inflammatory cytokine that women with PCOS are deficient in, adding to the deepest underlying cause of the condition.

Most concerning of all: Exposure to BPA changes the expression of genes during fetal development. The effects of this fetal exposure become apparent after puberty has begun, which has allowed it to remain hidden as a major causative force in PCOS. Puberty is the time when our hormones kick in for the reproductive phase of life. In PCOS, this simply doesn't happen in the typical way. Fueled by genes and environmental disruptors, reproductive activation is fundamentally changed. At puberty, there is a normal condition of insulin resistance that occurs, allowing a female to store fat, so she can prepare to reproduce. Unfortunately in PCOS, this insulin resistance uncovers the ovarian tendency to overproduce androgens and creates a vicious cycle between the pituitary gland and the ovaries. With underlying disruption previously caused by BPA, genetically susceptible women become far more likely to get stuck in the hormonal patterns of PCOS at puberty and often remain in this same pattern of insulin resistance, elevated LH, and androgen excess throughout their reproductive years.

Consider that when a female embryo is gestating in her mother's womb, her ovaries already have egg cells within them. Environmental exposure to toxins, such as BPA, during pregnancy can cause problems for not only the gestating fetus but also, if that fetus is female, for the fetus's ovaries and therefore her future children. That's right: Two generations can be affected by a single exposure.

Science confirms this. A recent study on rats found that exposure to even low levels of BPA during pregnancy induced PCOS in the offspring.[3]

The researchers timed the exposure to BPA for Day 8–15 of fetal development. This is when the rats' sexual organs were differentiating and is a crucial time in reproductive development.

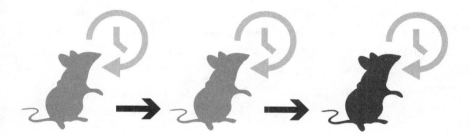

Figure 8-1: Rat Generations

The study also exposed pregnant rats to other endocrine-disrupting chemicals, including phthalates (found in plastics), pesticides, and the environmental pollutant dioxin. These are all chemicals that are prevalent in our environment. This single exposure triggered ovarian disease in future generations.

Even low doses of plastic exposure caused permanent PCOS-like changes in the ovaries for the second generation of rats. However, the strongest PCOS effect was actually seen in the third generation. Androgen levels were increased the most in this group. If this is the result of a single exposure to endocrine disruptors in pregnancy, imagine the impact of constant, chronic exposure, and the additive effects this will have on future generations. This is a key issue for not only our health as women but also that of our daughters (and sons, since BPA affects male reproductive development too) for generations to come. Although much of this relates to BPA, it is likely that the other xenoestrogens and endocrine-disrupting environmental chemicals have a similar action.

Types of Xenoestrogens, POPs, and EDCs

There are several types of xenoestrogens and endocrine disrupting chemicals that we are exposed to on a daily basis. Some of these include chemicals and plastics, skincare products, and pesticides as follows:

Chemicals and Plastics

- Bisphenol A
- Phthalates (found in plastics)
- PBDEs (flame retardants found in materials and furniture)
- PCBS (a product of manufacturing)
- Dioxin (an industrial pollutant)
- Perchlorate (an environmental contaminant found in our drinking water and much of our food supply)
- PFCs (used to make nonstick cookware and incredibly persistent in the human body and resistant to biodegration)
- Glycol ethers (found in cleaning products)
- Chlorine and bleach (the use of chlorine has been associated with the formation of compounds with BPA that have intense endocrine effects)

Skincare Products

- Parabens
- 4-MBC and benzophenone (sunscreens)
- Phalates (commonly found as diethyl phthalate [DEP])

Pesticides

- DDT (now illegal but still persists in the environment)
- Atrazine
- Organophosphate pesticides

Reducing Exposure to Endocrine Disruptors

Although it is true that endocrine disruptors are everywhere, there are ways we can reduce our exposure to them. Some things we can do include avoiding plastics in our food or when cooking, and being mindful of the beauty products and household cleaners we use, as follows:

Plastics

- Avoid using plastics and choose stainless steel, glass, or ceramics whenever possible. Most containers are now available in these materials, thankfully.
- Never microwave or heat up plastic containers containing food. Chemicals from the plastic will leach into your food.
- Avoid plastic wrap when possible, and never use it for heating food.
- Don't reuse plastic bottles. The BPA will leach out increasingly over time.
- Avoid canned foods or choose BPA-free cans.
- Do not use plastic water bottles that have heated up in the sun.
- Never use plastic sippy cups for children or plastic baby bottles. There are many glass and stainless steel options available.

Food and Cooking

- Whenever you can afford to do so, choose organic foods. This is particularly true of the infamous "dirty dozen," a list compiled each year by the Environmental Working Group of the twelve most heavily contaminated crops.
  - The list typically includes apples, celery, cherry tomatoes, cucumbers, grapes, peaches, nectarines, potatoes, snap peas, spinach, strawberries, sweet bell peppers, and kale/collards.
- Peel all nonorganic fruits and vegetables.
- Buy hormone-free, organic, grass-fed meats when possible.
- Choose organic, locally grown seasonal foods. These are often less contaminated, as they don't need additional preservation to stay fresh over a long transportation journey.
- Drink reverse osmosis water, as this can filter out most chemical residues.
- Avoid using nonstick cookware. Instead, choose ceramic, cast iron, stainless steel, or glass.

Beauty Products and Household Chemicals

- Avoid cosmetics and creams containing parabens.
- Avoid BHA and BHT. These are often used in moisturizers and makeup.
- Use chemical-free soaps and shampoos whenever possible.
- Avoid nail-care products with dibutyl phthalate.
- Check your beauty products on the Environmental Working Group to determine their potential for toxicity. The cosmetics database is a wonderful resource that is constantly updated. http://www.ewg.org/skindeep/
- Avoid using bleached coffee filters. These can result in a lifetime exposure to dioxin that creates risk for endocrine disruption.
- Avoid using pesticides in your garden or on your lawn.

Detoxification

Detoxification is a word that has a plethora of different meanings, including weight loss gimmicks; diets consisting of nothing but maple syrup, olive oil, and lemon juice; colon cleanses; juice cleanses; and the medical practice of detoxification in a hospital setting of a patient who has been exposed to dangerous chemicals. When it comes down to it, many commercial detoxification programs you'll see in stores or online don't provide much if any benefit. They are often simply composed of laxatives, fiber, and a restrictive diet.

It is unfortunate that the word detoxification now has an association with so many nonscientific practices, because it takes away from the fact that there is scientific validity to the process of detoxification. The most efficient system for detoxification is within our bodies already—the kidneys, liver, gastrointestinal tract, and immune system. These are typically capable of removing pollutants, drugs, and many other chemicals that affect our health. The human body is constantly in some state of detox, which is crucial to our survival.

Unlike the idea that we can somehow physically flush an organ out, which is not possible, particularly with any sort of vitamin or food regimen, I am suggesting something entirely different. I am offering a newer science that provides clear evidence that there are ways to help our bodies process environmental toxins. For example, there are specific nutrients and foods that can upregulate or induce the detoxification pathways in the liver that are known as Phase 1 and Phase 2, improving the rate and efficacy with which the liver can process and excrete a variety of toxins.

What I consider a detoxification program is to work to reduce your toxin exposure and increase foods and nutrients that induce both Phase 1 and Phase 2 detoxification processes, assisting the body in systematically processing and eliminating toxic compounds. In Phase 1, the liver uses oxygen to make toxins water soluble (many are fat soluble to begin with), so they can be easily excreted by the kidneys or liver. Many substances are not fully ready for excretion after Phase 1, when they are changed into an intermediate form that is actually harmful to the body. The toxin must be passed on to Phase 2 to be processed and eliminated. In Phase 2, these chemicals are combined with different compounds such as the amino acids cysteine, glycine, and methionine, and then finally excreted in the bile through the gallbladder.

Although again, most toxins can be effectively processed by our organs, research suggests that our exposure has increased at an alarming rate, with new substances added to our environment on a regular basis. Many people do need additional detoxification support due to increased exposure or increased demands on the liver. When more toxins must be processed, the need for the nutritional factors involved in their excretion increases as well.

Most importantly, we want to protect our tissues from toxins on a daily basis, since exposure is so constant. For example, N-acetyl cysteine, which benefits women with respect to insulin resistance and inflammation, can play a dual role, as it aids in detoxification. So can drinking enough water, eating foods that are rich in cofactors required by the liver, and including plenty of fiber to ensure regular bowel movements, as toxins are also excreted in the stool.

Often, when embarking on a new nutrition plan for PCOS, it is helpful to view the first two to four weeks as a detox (depending on your level of exposure to toxins or if lifestyle permits a shorter versus longer detox) where you remove sugars, processed foods, and dairy strictly from your diet for a given time. This not only gives your body and brain a reset when it comes to food habits and taste preferences, but it also helps to set up new lifestyle patterns as well.

During this period of time, it may be helpful to add specific support for detoxification. These steps can include—

- Strict avoidance of alcohol, unnecessary over-the-counter medications, and foods with high pesticide content that create an extra burden for your liver.

- Drink plenty of water to prevent dehydration and ensure good excretion through the kidneys.

- Support for Phase 1 detoxification can include B complex vitamins, vitamin C, and glutathione, which can be increased in the liver by the herb milk thistle.[4]

- Support for Phase 2 detoxification, which includes glycine, N-acetyl cysteine (NAC), curcumin, and B vitamins.[5]
- Support the additional needs of Phase 2 detoxification with sulphur-rich foods such as broccoli, kale, brussels sprouts, onions, and garlic.[6,7]
- Increase dietary fiber to ensure regular bowel movements, as toxic compounds are excreted through the gallbladder into the intestines. An optimal source of fiber for women with PCOS is vegetables. Great sources of fiber include cabbage, celery, broccoli, collards, root vegetables like carrots and squash, and leafy green vegetables like collards, kale, Swiss chard, and bok choy. These vegetables are rich in insoluble fiber that helps to recycle bile and cholesterol and improve bowel regularity.

Detoxification is a continuous process, because we are always being exposed to environmental toxins. It is an excellent idea to increase the foods listed here on a daily basis to help ensure sufficiency of the required cofactors for both Phase 1 and Phase 2. This will allow our natural detoxification system to better manage toxins, minimizing the exposure we receive to harmful chemicals within our bodies.

Endocrine disruptors are powerful chemicals that can scramble our hormonal messages from their most basic origins. Chronic exposure to these compounds, particularly in pregnant women, unmasks and turns on the genes for PCOS that will be seen at the time of puberty when the hormones activate. This effect persists and compounds through generations. Although it is a challenge to actually change the effect of endocrine disruptors, awareness is critical. These compounds continue to be added to not only our environment but also to our bodies and to those of our children and future generations.

Chapter 9

STEP 8. EAT A BALANCED DIET

Don't eat anything your great-grandmother wouldn't recognize as food.
—MICHAEL POLLAN

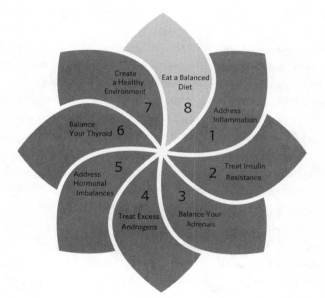

In my clinic, we've tried many different types of nutritional plans for women with PCOS over the years. One thing I've learned is that no one diet program works for everyone with PCOS. As we've seen by looking intensively at each of the factors involved, we are all unique. So, although I'll spell the recommended nutritional program out here, there may be some adjustments that you'll need to make. First of all, I'll cover what to eat, as well as macronutrients and meal composition, as sometimes it's a lot harder to know what you *should* eat, rather than what you shouldn't. Then, I'll cover what to avoid.

The Importance of Glucose and Insulin

We've already talked about insulin resistance in detail, and it's important to understand that insulin isn't, in general, a bad thing. Insulin takes sugar from the bloodstream and helps it to enter the cells to be used for energy or to be stored. It's like a key that opens the lock to our cells.

It also stops glucose from being released by the liver into the bloodstream. We don't want to view insulin as the enemy. It's a very important hormone needed for survival. However, for women with PCOS, it's also something that we know aggravates our condition hormonally.

Numerous studies show that elevated insulin levels are caused by a combination of genetics, obesity, and a variety of other factors. One thing is clear: Being of an increased weight causes large amounts of insulin to be released, creating insulin resistance. There are numerous cultures that consume a lot of carbohydrates, and yet people from these cultures can be of average weight or lean. This occurs because the overall composition of the diet, lifestyle, and genetics support health and leanness. So, I don't want to give anyone the impression that carbohydrates are in any way "bad." In this book, we are addressing PCOS, which has its own set of unique nutritional considerations. There is a population of people who are genetically insulin resistant and are predisposed to type 2 diabetes. For these individuals, consuming foods that spike insulin contributes to their pathology of insulin resistance. Those with PCOS are also insulin resistant. High insulin levels aggravate our insulin-sensitive ovaries and cause them to make testosterone, stalling ovulation and blocking the hormonal cycles. When insulin may be very high already, as is the case in insulin-resistant women with PCOS, we certainly don't want to add fuel to the fire.

First, let's talk about a few important concepts: the glycemic index, the glycemic load, and the food insulin index. Then we will get to a new concept—what might very well be one of the best new methods for women with PCOS who want to increase insulin sensitivity.

Carbohydrates and the Glycemic Index

Let's talk more about carbohydrates now. As PCOS is so closely linked to insulin resistance and diabetes, this is a much talked about subject. We all have heard that we should limit our carbohydrates and keep the foods that we eat lower on the glycemic index. This is true for many women. However, we know so much more now due to new information on insulin and how it works in our bodies that we have to address other factors as well.

The glycemic index, which you've probably heard of, is a marker of how quickly a food breaks down into sugar within the bloodstream. It's the measurement of how much a food with 50 grams of carbohydrates raises blood sugar over two hours, compared to how much 50 grams of glucose would. The closer to 100, the closer to pure sugar. This has been a popular concept in creating a healthy diet for women with PCOS.

Although the glycemic index has been so widely used, I think there are some other factors to consider in finding the best diet for PCOS. The glycemic index only measures blood glucose rise due to the consumption of carbohydrates and doesn't take into account the effect of any of the other nutrients on our metabolic health, most especially on that of insulin—clearly an important factor for women with PCOS.

Although it's popularly thought that only carbohydrates cause the secretion of insulin, proteins also cause significant insulin release. So the glycemic index falls short in this area. Other areas that the glycemic index misses are that its measurement is for 50 grams of a food. And as we know, we eat different serving sizes based on the type of food we consume. For example, 50 grams of jellybeans is very different in size than 50 grams of watermelon.

The glycemic load is what accounts for the quantity consumed when referring to the glycemic index. Basically, it's the amount of food eaten, multiplied by the glycemic index of the food. So our watermelon would have a low glycemic load, whereas jellybeans would have a high glycemic load. Eating very few jellybeans would raise your blood sugar quite a bit. To get the same rise in blood sugar from watermelon, you would need to eat quite a bit of watermelon. To give you an idea of why this is important, consider the following: If you choose a food that is moderate on the glycemic index and you eat a large quantity of it, you are still increasing the load of carbohydrates to be processed by the body. That being said, although the glycemic load can be helpful when formulating nutritional plans for women with PCOS, it has some limitations. This is because it does not measure the insulin production for each food. And for us, this is the most important thing.

Satiety Index

Here's another important consideration. There are certain foods that are much more filling than others. In fact, this seems to be completely independent of effects on insulin or blood sugar. A measurement called the satiety index was created in the mid-nineties by researcher Dr. Susanna Holt. It charts which foods stave off hunger the best by measuring how full people feel from consuming the same number of calories of different foods. It doesn't measure anything about nutritional content. Instead, it measures how full a food can keep you feeling. As such, this index is really most helpful for those who are trying to lose weight or maintain weight loss. The factors that help a food come up high on the satiety index include water content, fiber, and protein. Interestingly, potatoes, one of the highest foods on the glycemic index, came in tops on the satiety index!

The satiety index has limits. For example, it only contains thirty-eight foods. However if you look at nutritiondata.self.com, there's a similar index called the Fullness Factor™. This scale has calculated the ability of a food to create fullness based on the nutrient composition and is thought to be quite accurate overall. It gives each food a satiety rank based on how filling it is per calorie.

Another benefit of this scale is that it allows you to create mixed meals and then generate an overall fullness factor for the whole meal. I do like using this factor, especially for women who would like to lose weight. It definitely makes weight loss much easier when you feel satisfied after eating.

The Food Insulin Index and Insulin Counting

Now I would like to cover what I consider to be the single best way to regulate insulin secretion after meals. This is a new concept that you may not have even heard of, but I think it's important. This concept was introduced in 1997 by a group of diabetes researchers associated with the University of Sydney, Australia. This is the same group of people, including the esteemed Dr. Jennie Brand-Miller, who are considered to be the world's foremost experts on the glycemic index and are some of the most brilliant researchers in the field of diabetes.

The researchers began by testing thirty-eight foods in healthy volunteers to see how much these foods raised blood insulin after consuming them. They found the foods that raised blood glucose the most (foods high on the glycemic index) also raised blood insulin levels.[1] They named this index the food insulin index (FII), which is similar to the glycemic index, but instead of measuring blood glucose responses after eating a specific food, it measures how much insulin your body secretes instead.

Since elevations in blood sugar cause our pancreas to secrete insulin, it makes sense that foods high on the glycemic index are also high on the insulin index. The researchers at the University of Sydney also found something else that was remarkably interesting: Protein-rich foods were capable of raising insulin responses in a way that was disproportionately high compared to their effects on blood sugar. We know that proteins are exceptionally low on the glycemic index, so it was quite interesting to see that they stimulate the release of insulin. This information has the potential to change the clinical practice of diabetes management.

First, I want to be very clear that PCOS is different than diabetes—it is a condition of insulin resistance and not of hyperglycemia. So, although we do want to maintain blood sugar control, controlling insulin resistance is the main focus. That is why this new index, which is showing great promise for diabetes, may in fact be the most well-suited program for women with PCOS.

In 2011, the FII was increased to include around 120 foods.[2] In 2014, researcher Kirstine Bell produced a brilliant PhD thesis, "Clinical Application of the Food

Table 9-1: A Satiety Index of Common Foods

FOOD	SATIETY INDEX
Bone broth (estimated)	350% +
Non-starchy vegetables (estimated)	350% +
Potatoes, boiled	323%
Fish and chicken (estimated)	225%
Oranges	202%
Apples	197%
Beef	176%
Grapes	162%
Eggs	150%
White rice	138%
Brown rice	132%
White pasta	119%
Bananas	118%
White bread	100%
Potato chips	91%
Yogurt	88%
Peanuts	84%
Chocolate bar	70%
Croissant	47%

All foods are compared to white bread, which is designated a satiety index of 100. The higher the satiety index, the more satisfying the food is.

Non-starchy vegetables, although not directly tested in the source of this study (though estimated in other indices that can't be directly compared), are very high on the satiety index. They are exceptionally filling per calorie and would be at the top of this list.

Sources:

Holt SH, Miller JC, Petocz P, Farmakalidis E. A satiety index of common foods. *Eur J Clin Nutr.* 1995; 49(9):675-690.

Insulin Index to Diabetes Mellitus," that increased this list by another twenty-six foods and tested the concept in clinical practice. The results were fascinating. Using the FII provided even better control of diabetes than the current gold standard, which is carbohydrate counting. She also detailed a new idea that could be put into clinical practice. This idea is known as food insulin demand (FID). FID is a measurement of the insulin response to a given food, taking into account the FII of the food and, most importantly, how many calories of the food are consumed.

I believe that the best marker you can use to track how foods affect your insulin is the FID, because it accounts for different macronutrients, not just carbohydrates. Most of all, it accounts for the rise in insulin after eating, which is a concern for most women with PCOS. Even better, it accounts for how many calories of insulin-spiking foods that you are consuming, providing, in my opinion, the most comprehensive way to track the effects of diet on insulin in our bodies.

As the insulin index of a food is calculated for 239 calories of any given food, the FID is relatively easy to calculate. FID = calories × the FII of the food item/239 calories. I do want to note, however, that just because protein raises insulin levels does not mean you should avoid it.

One of insulin's jobs is to send amino acids into our muscle tissue, so it makes sense that protein-rich foods would increase insulin, but protein doesn't increase blood sugar like carbohydrates do. Protein-rich foods are high on the insulin index, yet low on the glycemic index.

Glucagon

That's where glucagon comes in. Glucagon tells the liver to release glucose into the bloodstream when the blood sugar becomes low, which keeps your blood sugar level stable. When you eat high-protein foods, insulin and glucagon are released. When you eat high-carbohydrate foods, only insulin is released.

Glucagon does increase satiety (fullness), which may partly explain the benefits of high-protein diets on weight loss. Glucagon also keeps the blood sugar quite stable after the consumption of protein, which is beneficial. Another factor in support of eating protein is that the amino acid leucine acts in the brain on special compounds known as the mechanistic target of rapamycin (mTOR) and AMP-activated protein kinase (AMPK). These are the cells' way of sensing energy, and this pathway seems to be important in the ability of high-protein diets to improve weight loss, increase muscle mass, and reduce fat mass.

So overall, eating protein is exceptionally beneficial. However, we should try to stick more to proteins that are lower in FID whenever possible. Beef has a much higher FID than chicken, for example. This is related to the specific amino acid composition of each type of protein.

Note: This is for around 239 calories of each food as shown in Table 9-2. Remember that 239 calories of a vegetable like cauliflower would come to a much larger amount than 239 calories of pasta. This is why, when choosing foods, the food insulin demand is the more accurate way of measuring a food's impact on your insulin levels: It not only accounts for the food's ability to increase insulin but also for the amount you are consuming.

Table 9-2: The Food Insulin Index and Food Insulin Demand for Some Common Foods

	FOOD INSULIN INDEX FOR 239 CALORIES (1000KJ)	SERVING SIZE	FOOD INSULIN DEMAND FOR TYPICAL SERVING
Proteins			
Roast chicken	17	130 grams	20
Grilled lean beef steak	37	130 grams	30
Grilled lamb fillet	21	130 grams	20
White fish (ling cod)	43	130 grams	17
Tuna in oil, drained	16	80 grams	9
Poached eggs	23	2 large (100 g)	14
Shrimp	21	7 shrimp (98 g)	9
Short cut bacon	9	2 slices (72 g)	6
Navy beans	23	½ cup	11
Whey (estimated)	138.7	28 grams	59
Fats			
Walnuts	5	¼ cup	4
Peanuts	15	¼ cup	12
Peanut butter	11	1 tbsp	4
Olive oil	3	1 tbsp	2
Avocado	4	¼ (50 g)	2
Carbohydrate Rich Foods			
Boiled potatoes	88	1 medium (150 g)	36
White rice (estimated)	53	1 cup	46
Whole grain pasta	29	1 cup	20
Brown rice	45	1 cup	49
Butternut squash	77	1 cup (205 g)	37
White bread	73	2 slices	52
Sweet potato	96	1 small (120 g)	37

continued on next page

	FOOD INSULIN INDEX FOR 239 CALORIES (1000KJ)	SERVING SIZE	FOOD INSULIN DEMAND FOR TYPICAL SERVING
Pancakes	110	1–100g pancakes	83
Reduced-fat blueberry muffin	69	1 large muffin (170 g)	116
Fruit			
Banana	59	1 medium (118 g)	25
Grapes	60	12 grapes (120 g)	18
Oranges	44	1 medium (230 g)	11
*Apple (Red Delicious)	43	1 medium (140 g)	15
*Honeydew melon	93	1 slice (125 g)	16
*Peach	39	1 medium (150 g)	10
Dairy			
Low fat fruit yogurt	84	175 gram container	57
Plain yogurt	46	175 gram container	38
Skim milk	60	250 ml	21
Cheddar cheese		1 slice (25 g)	14
Low fat cottage cheese		1 cup (240 g)	42
Vegetables			
Green peas—steamed	18	1 cup	16
Broccoli—steamed	29	1 cup	3
Cauliflower—steamed	48	1 cup	6
Carrots—steamed	44	1 cup	9

* Weights are for edible portion only.

Values sourced and/or estimated from Nilsson M., Stenberg M., Frid A. H., Holst J. J., Bjorck I. M. 2004. "Glycemia and Insulinemia in Healthy Subjects after Lactose-Equivalent Meals of Milk and Other Food Proteins: The Role Of Plasma Amino Acids and Incretins." *American Journal of Clinical Nutrition*. 80 (5):1246–1253.

To make things very simple, I have also created an easy to use "insulin count" for you. This is an approximation and is based on the insulin index and FOD, but it makes it easy to calculate the insulin effect of commonly eaten foods and quantities on your metabolic health.

Only some foods have been tested for their FII so far, so some of the foods listed in Table 9-3 are approximations based on other similar foods or their individual components. You can also create your own insulin count of mixed foods by adding together their components. If you visit my website at http://drfionand.com/insulin-count, you'll find this table as well as a calculator that will help you with this. In time, as more foods are tested, we will be able to adjust these counts with more accuracy.

Table 9-3: Insulin Count of Recommended Foods for Women with PCOS

	SERVING SIZE	INSULIN COUNT
Proteins		
Roast chicken/turkey	130 grams	20
Lean beef steak	130 grams	30
White fish	130 grams	17
Beans, lentils, chickpeas, hummus	130 grams ½ cup	11 (estimated)
Eggs	2 large	14
Shrimp	7 shrimp (98 g)	9
Bacon/back bacon	2 slices	6
Lamb or pork	130 grams	20
Whey protein powder	25 grams	53 (estimated)
Vegan protein powder	25 grams	32 (estimated)
Fats and Oils		
Nuts and seeds	1 ounce (closed handful)	4 (estimated)
Olive oil and other oils	1 tbsp	1.5
Avocado and guacamole	½ medium or 70 grams	3
Nut butters	1 tbsp	5 (estimated)
Carbohydrates		
Boiled potatoes	1 medium (150 g)	36
White rice	1 cup	46
Whole grain quinoa pastas	1 cup	20
Brown rice	1 cup	49

continued on next page

	SERVING SIZE	INSULIN COUNT
Pumpkin and squash	1 cup (205 g)	37
Almond flour muffin	1 small	10 (estimated)
Fruit		
Banana	1 medium	25
Grapes	1 cup	15
Oranges and citrus	1 medium	11
Apples, pears	1 medium	15
Melons	1 cup	23
Peaches	1 medium	10
Berries	1 cup	2 (estimated)
Dairy Substitutes		
Unsweetened almond or cashew milk	1 cup	< 2 (estimated)
Unsweetened coconut milk	1 cup	< 3 (estimated)
Vegetables		
Cooked broccoli and cauliflower	1 cup	4
Carrots	1 cup	9
Green peas	1 cup	18
All other non-starchy raw and cooked vegetables	1 cup	2 (estimated)

Adapted and estimated from Bao et al., 2011; Holt, Miller, and Petocz, 1997; and K. Bell 1968.

You should also consider that raw vegetables, in addition to having a low insulin count, are high on the satiety index, so if you are feeling hungry, try adding more salad to each meal.

You may also have noticed that protein powders can be quite high on the insulin index—in particular, whey protein. This is because of the large amount of branched chain amino acids that are in whey. These amino acids can easily and quickly enter the bloodstream. One of the best times to use a protein powder such as whey is directly after working out, particularly after weight training. This way, the spike in insulin is used to drive amino acids into the muscle cells for building and repairing tissue. Enjoy a starch, like a few chunks of steamed or baked sweet potato, with your protein powder post-workout and you're set!

What to Eat and What Not to Eat

Now that we've got the macronutrients down and the effects of different types of food on our insulin responses, I want to talk about food quality and which categories and types of foods are best to eat and avoid for women with PCOS.

Foods to Include

There are a variety of healthy food choices you can make if you have PCOS. The foods in this section are those you can include in your diet.

Vegetables

It goes without saying that the vast majority of what you eat should be plants. Plant foods are jam-packed with an exceptionally wide variety of nutrients, including vitamins, minerals, and phytonutrients, as well as both soluble and insoluble fibers. All of these are preventive for the vast majority of diseases that humanity suffers from today. Most of all, study after study highlights their benefits in the prevention of type 2 diabetes, cardiovascular disease, cancer, and their ability to improve metabolic health. For optimal health, you should include vegetables with a wide variety of colors and focus primarily on non-starchy vegetables.

Non-Starchy Vegetables

Most non-starchy vegetables are given the green light, meaning you can eat plenty of these every day. They are rich in fiber, water, numerous vitamins and minerals, and they have a high satiety index and low insulin/glycemic indices. Following are some examples of non-starchy vegetables. You should be having at least half a large dinner plate of these with every meal:

- Raw, leafy greens, including bitter salad greens, romaine lettuce, dandelion greens, arugula greens, spinach, and baby kale
- Cooked leafy greens, including Swiss chard, kale, spinach, and collard greens
- Brussels sprouts, broccoli, bok choy, cabbage, and cauliflower
- Carrots
- Green and French beans
- Mushrooms of all varieties

- Sprouts, including alfalfa, mung bean, and broccoli
- Artichokes
- Bell peppers
- Eggplant
- Sea vegetables, such as nori and wakame
- Cucumbers
- Celery
- Onions and garlic

Starchy Vegetables

Rather than deriving carbohydrates from grains, starchy vegetables are a better choice because they do not contain irritants or phytates that decrease nutrient absorption. If you are exercising, you'll need more carbohydrates to fuel your workouts and your recovery.

Starchy vegetables can have a higher glycemic index and have higher carbohydrate loads than non-starchy vegetables, so smaller amounts should be consumed. To make meal prep easier, I often chop and freeze starchy vegetables for the week and use them as needed for meals. Some examples include—

- Parsnips. These "white carrots" are a nutritious carbohydrate source. They can be baked in the oven to create delicious parsnip French fries.
- Squash, including acorn, butternut, spaghetti, and pumpkin, are all nutrient-dense sources of lower glycemic index carbohydrates. They are rich in fiber, vitamins, and minerals.
- Sweet potatoes. These are one of the most famous healthy starchy vegetables. Sweet potatoes are easy to digest, delicious, and high in fiber and nutrition. While they are high on the insulin count, they are also very filling.
- White potato. White potatoes are easy to digest and nutritious and need not be eliminated from the diet. They are the highest rated food on the satiety index, so it's OK to enjoy them once in a while as part of a balanced meal.
- Beets. A nutritional powerhouse, beets are an excellent source of nutrient-dense carbohydrates. Added to a smoothie, or baked as a side dish with your dinner, these will provide antioxidants, vitamins, and minerals as well as fuel for your body.

Fruits

Fruits are an excellent source of fiber, vitamins, and minerals and are one of the main sources of carbohydrates that should be included in a diet for PCOS. They are also a healthy option you can take quickly on the go. As fruits do contain significant amounts of natural sugars, it's best to choose the lowest sugar fruits as a general rule. Other fruits can also be enjoyed if the quantities are kept in check.

The lowest sugar content fruits are—

- Avocados*
- Tomatoes*
- Lemons and limes
- Raspberries
- Blackberries
- Blueberries
- Strawberries
- Cranberries
- Rhubarb
- Papaya
- Grapefruit

*Although not thought of as a fruit, these are an amazingly low-insulin index choice and should be eaten regularly.

Medium-sugar fruits include—
- Cantaloupe
- Honeydew
- Apricots
- Apples
- Oranges
- Pears
- Kiwi
- Plums
- Pineapple

High-sugar fruits include—

- Cherries
- Mangos
- Dates
- Figs
- Grapes
- Pomegranate
- Bananas**

**If they are ripe. If they are unripe, they are much lower in sugar.

Oils

Oils are an important part of a healthy diet. We were all taught that fat was bad during the low-fat diet phases of the 1990s and 2000s. Recently, this has been completely debunked. Fats can be and are good for you. It's really the type of fat that makes the difference.

When it comes to vegetable oils, you'll want to choose them carefully. The reason for this is that vegetable oils are made of primarily unsaturated fats, which means they have delicate bonds within their structure that are sensitive and can be broken down rather easily. There are two major types of unsaturated fats: polyunsaturated and monounsaturated. Polyunsaturated fats, just as the name suggests, have multiple delicate bonds within them. Monounsaturated fats have only one delicate bond within. Because of these extra delicate bonds, polyunsaturated fats are more vulnerable to damage and must be treated with more care. We all have learned that polyunsaturated fats are good for us, and they actually are a very healthy part of our diet, particularly those of the omega-3 variety.

The main issue is that the vast majority of polyunsaturated fats that we consume have been heavily processed. They have also been exposed to heat, chemicals, and light during processing, causing the bonds to break down within the fats. What happens when the bonds break down? The fat changes form into a type of fat known as lipid peroxide, which is quite harmful.

The vegetable oils that are the most concerning are canola oil, sunflower oil, corn oil, safflower oil, and cottonseed oil. These oils are mass-produced and treated with chemicals and heats that damage the very nature of the oil. The oil is extracted from the seed with chemical solvents. In addition, once you take this oil and use it to cook your food, you are heating it up even more, increasing the toxic potential of the oil.

The other negative with many of these oils is that they contain large amounts of omega-6 fatty acids. Too many omega-6 fatty acids can increase inflammation, and it is very difficult to keep the levels of these in your diet in check, since they are present in so many foods.

It's also important to know that our cell membranes are made up of fatty acids. Polyunsaturated fatty acids can be good for our cell membranes, as are saturated fatty acids. Together, these two types of fatty acids give our cell membranes fluidity. This helps with the function of every cell in the body. However, if polyunsaturated fatty acid is exposed to heat or oxygen, it turns into lipid peroxide, which can damage the cell membranes and also the DNA within our cells. Lipid peroxides can also damage the phospholipids in the cell membrane, eventually poking holes in our cells, allowing free radicals to enter into our cells and damage them.

In addition to lipid peroxides, we all know that trans fats are unhealthy, as they are associated with multiple diseases, including cardiovascular disease and cancer. What isn't known is that vegetable oils contain trans fats. Research has found that many commonly sold vegetable oils contain these fats, presumably because of the way they are processed. Trans fats don't exist in nature; they are the result of the processing of oils. When incorporated into cell membranes, a variety of different dysfunction occurs.

When it comes to vegetable oils, the best are avocado oil, extra virgin olive oil, and coconut oil. Avocado oil and extra virgin olive oil contain monounsaturated fats and are far more stable than the polyunsaturated oils. They appear to be stable under very low-heat cooking. Olive oil, in particular, has been researched extensively and has many health benefits. I recommend using only these as your sources of liquid vegetable oils.

As cooking oil for very hot temperatures, extra virgin coconut oil is the best choice. Being comprised of saturated fat, it's exceptionally stable when heated and when stored. When it comes to avoiding the coconut flavor in your cooking, there is the option of expeller-pressed organic coconut oil, which is available at most organic grocery stores. This doesn't have as many health benefits as extra virgin coconut oil, but it is still a good choice when you want to avoid coconut flavor in your food.

Another option for high-temperature cooking is clarified butter, also known as ghee. Ghee, particularly when organic and taken from grass-fed cows, has a variety of health benefits and contains a compound known as butyrate, which is beneficial for intestinal health. As much of the milk solids are removed, it does not have the insulin spiking effects that other dairy products have.

That being said, since hormones are always concentrated in the fat portion of dairy, always choose organic and don't overdo it.

I'm also going to include avocado in the oils section even though it is a fruit, as it contains wonderful fats. Adding a quarter of an avocado to a meal will make you feel fuller longer and provide a wonderful source of nutrition to your diet.

Meats

Meats, including fish, poultry, red meats, and game, can be an excellent source of protein and micronutrients for women with PCOS. In addition to protein, meats contain a variety of vitamins, minerals, and omega-3 fatty acids that provide dense nutrition. It's helpful if you can afford organic and especially pastured or grass-fed meats, as they have improved nutritional composition and less toxicity.

Fish

Fish have gotten a bad rap lately due to toxicity; however, they are an excellent source of nutrition. And although they do increase insulin to some degree, like all proteins, they have so many wonderful nutritional benefits and they should definitely be included in the PCOS-friendly diet. High in omega-3 fatty acids, protein, and vitamins A, D, and magnesium, they are an excellent source of lean protein to add to a meal. There are two main contaminants to look out for in fish: mercury and PCB. However, fish is such a healthy food that the benefits often outweigh the risk of contamination, especially if you choose your fish carefully.

Mercury is one of the most toxic metals to the human body. As such, this should be our primary concern when it comes to choosing fish. Large, predatory fish are particularly likely to concentrate mercury in their tissues. As all fish do contain some mercury, when larger fish eat smaller fish, they accumulate more of it in their bodies over time. As mercury comes primarily from industrial contamination, fish that are caught near a coast or freshwater where there is a human population are also more likely to be contaminated.

The fish that are highest in mercury include—

- Shark
- Swordfish
- Marlin
- Tuna
- King mackerel
- Grouper

Fish that are generally lower in mercury include—

- Wild Alaska salmon
- Sardines
- Anchovies
- Atlantic pollock
- Atlantic mackerel
- Shrimp
- Catfish
- Crab
- Crawfish
- Mussels
- Sockeye salmon
- Line caught (longline) albacore yellowfin tuna

To learn more about mercury levels in fish, there is an excellent website located at http://seafood.edf.org/seafood-health-alerts. The Environmental Defense Fund also keeps an excellent updated database on the mercury content in fish.

Many people ask about farmed versus wild salmon. My opinion on salmon is that if you can get it, wild Alaska or sockeye salmon are by far your best bet. Wild salmon has a better fatty acid profile than farmed salmon, as farmed salmon are fed a different diet with the goal of fattening up the fish. The main concern with farmed salmon is that they do contain much higher levels of PCBs when compared to wild salmon.[3]

If you can afford it, wild Alaska salmon is the best choice. Fortunately, most canned salmon is wild Alaska or sockeye, which are excellent healthy and affordable choices. Once in a while, however, farmed salmon can be included in your diet, particularly if you are replacing less healthy choices with it, such as when going out for dinner or at a friend's home. If you are pregnant, breastfeeding, or trying to conceive, however, I would avoid farmed salmon.

In addition to mercury, the levels of PCB and other contaminants in fish may vary greatly, depending on where the fish are caught. PCBs are particularly concerning for women in their childbearing years, as they can affect the development of the fetus. In addition, increased PCBs have been linked to developmental problems in children. Fish that tend to be the highest in PCBs are those that reside near industrial areas and are bottom feeders. These include wild-striped bass, bluefish, American eel, and sea trout.

Poultry

Chicken, turkey, Cornish hen, pheasant, and other poultry are an excellent source of lean protein for women with PCOS. They are high in niacin, selenium, and vitamin B6. It is optimal to access pastured poultry from a farmer if you can, due to toxicity concerns detailed below—organic is also a good choice. If you only have access to conventional poultry, be sure to remove the fat before cooking. Poultry, on the whole, has a lower insulin index for a protein-rich food, yet it is highly satisfying and so is helpful for those who are more insulin resistant and want to lose weight. If you get a pastured chicken, be sure to save the bones and make bone broth—you'll find instructions on how to make this healing, nourishing food in the recipes appendix.

Bone broth can be made from any type of bone—many women find it an excellent addition to breakfast, as a filling, nutritious, and delicious start to the day. Some women also have a cup with dinner. As you can imagine, bone broth is high on the satiety index, given its low energy density, but it also is packed with nutrients. Since bone broth is often cooked for many hours with herbs and vegetables, it contains a variety of vitamins and minerals. In addition, when a bone is cooked for a long period of time, as in bone broth, it becomes rich in amino acids like proline and glycine. Glycine in particular is beneficial, as glucose regulation, insulin sensitivity, and the production of the main intracellular antioxidant, glutathione, rely on it.

Red Meat

Red meat, including beef, lamb, and pork, definitely has excellent nutritional value. It has a good deal of protein and is a rich source of many nutrients, including B vitamins, iron, zinc, selenium, copper, and potassium. Beef and lamb, in particular, are the best sources of zinc, B vitamins, and iron. Pork only offers modest amounts of these.

We talked about certain amino acids being more insulinogenic than others. Well, how does this relate to meats? There are, in fact, meats that are better for women with PCOS to consume. Beef is quite high on the insulin index, so it is the least recommended. If you do consume red meat, you should be aware of the quantity and that, if you are insulin counting, you get less quantity-wise for red meat than you do for poultry. Another major concern for women with PCOS is that red meat, like dairy, contains estrogen, so for that reason, as well, it should be consumed only in moderation.[4]

When it comes to consuming red meats, you'll also want to avoid high-heat cooking. Carcinogenic byproducts are created when red meats are heated at high temperatures and through fermentation by the gut microbiome. These toxic products include heterocyclic amines and polyaromatic hydrocarbons (PAH). So, when cooking animal proteins, use low heat whenever possible.

Grass-fed, organic meats are the best choice for beef. Not only do they contain lower amounts of contaminants, such as medications or hormones, they also provide better nutrition. These animals graze on grass, and, as such, their tissues are quite different composition-wise. Animals that are grass fed have more omega-3 fatty acids and micronutrients like vitamin E, zinc, and carotenoids.[5, 6] Another popular red meat is bison, which is becoming increasingly available on the market, offering another more natural alternative to conventional beef.

It is unfortunate that in North America, artificial hormones are used on livestock to increase their growth. In the US, recombinant bovine somatotropin (rBST), also known as rBGH, causes an increase in another growth hormone, IGF-1, in treated cows. Some studies have associated risk for breast, colon, and prostate cancer with increased serum levels of IGF-1.[7, 8, 9] In addition, cows given rBGH are more prone to infection of their udders, known as mastitis, resulting in an increased need for antibiotics.

Another consideration is that in most modern feedlots where animals are raised, the conditions are unsanitary, and low-dose antibiotics are routinely given to the animals to prevent infection. Antibiotics are also used to increase the growth rates of the animals. Surprisingly, a survey from John Hopkins's Center found that eighty percent of all antibiotics sold were for use on livestock and poultry.[10]

Pesticide residues also accumulate in the tissues of animals. Dioxins are one of the most concerning environmental toxins and have been linked to cancer, reproductive problems, cardiovascular disease, and diabetes. It is thought that ninety percent of human exposure to dioxins comes from animal fats, fish, and shellfish.

If you can locate a farmer who sells meat in your area, this is often the best option, as you can inquire about their farming practices. Many farms with ethical, organic practices will provide plenty of information on their websites. Local farmers markets are also good places to source quality meats directly from the farmer. Many small farms offer bulk purchasing of meats, which can make it more affordable to buy quality meats. Another excellent option is community-supported agriculture (CSA). In this situation, you pay a one-time fee to support the farmer each season, and then you receive a biweekly or monthly portion of meat fresh from the farm. The same can be done with organic produce, so if you want to have regular access to more affordable quality food and support local farmers this is a great option.

When consuming meats—

- Choose grass-fed beef, pastured pork, and organic free-range or pastured chicken, particularly from a farmer who you know uses good farming practices.

- If you're not able to obtain organic or grass-fed meats, buy the leanest cuts that you can, remove all of the visible fat, and make the consumption of red meat a rare occurrence, focusing more on poultry and seafood.

- As much of the contamination in meat is found in the fat, removing it will help you to minimize the consumption of unwanted toxins.

- When grilling meats, remove the fat first to reduce the formation of polyaromatic cyclic hydrocarbons(PAH), a cancer-causing compound.

- Avoid charring or cooking red meats at high temperatures to avoid formation of PAH.

- Marinate meats first with rosemary and/or lemon juice, as this reduces the formation of carcinogenic compounds.

Eggs

Eggs are one of my favorite foods for women with PCOS. They include a wonderful nutrient profile, including folate, vitamin A, vitamin B2, vitamin B12, choline, and selenium. In addition, they contain an amazing amount of protein for a small amount of calories and are filling and satisfying. A boiled egg or two packed with your lunch or for a breakfast on the go can prevent you from making poor food choices when you are out. Even better, chickens that are fed quality feed, such as those that are pastured (the chickens run free eating insects and feed), as well as organic eggs, have an excellent fatty acid profile and an even better nutritional value.

So what about cholesterol? I get this question often, as women with PCOS are more at risk for high cholesterol, which is an important issue for us. I'll just let you know for certain that eating eggs does not increase your cholesterol, unless you have a rare form of familial hypercholesterolemia. Your liver manufacturers cholesterol from the foods that you eat, and when you eat eggs, your liver will not make as much as it would normally. For a small percentage of people, eating eggs will mildly raise their total and LDL cholesterol, but for the vast majority of people, eggs raise the good HDL cholesterol. In addition, it appears that eggs increase the LDL cholesterol into a subtype called large LDL. It's the small, dense LDL that is linked most to heart disease. If you are following the healthy diet recommendations in this chapter, you should see improvements in your cholesterol panel, despite eating eggs on a regular basis. What you eat and your level of exercise will determine your cholesterol levels.

Nuts and Seeds

Nuts and seeds are excellent sources of nutrition. They contain healthy fats, protein, vitamins, and minerals, such as vitamin E and magnesium, and best of all, they are satiating. They do contain phytates, so they should not be consumed with each meal.

The other downside of nuts and seeds is that they have a very high caloric density. It's very easy to eat handfuls of nuts, and before you know it, you will have consumed a thousand calories. As such, I often recommend measuring nuts and seeds and placing them on a plate before consuming them. As is the case with legumes, sprouting or soaking nuts and seeds will reduce the phytate concentration. Quinoa, although thought of as a grain, is actually a seed. It's something that I recommend in moderation also, and, if possible, sprouted to reduce phytate concentration.

The most nutrient dense nuts and seeds are—

- Almonds
- Pecans
- Cashews
- Macadamia nuts
- Brazil nuts
- Pistachios
- Pumpkin seeds
- Sunflower seeds
- Walnuts

Legumes

Legumes include beans, chickpeas, lentils, and peanuts and are what I would consider a nutritional grey area. Legumes do contain significant amounts of phytic acid and may inhibit the absorption of nutrients. That being said, legumes can be an excellent source of fiber, vitamins, and minerals, so I often tell patients that legumes are one of those areas for which you have to make an individual choice. If you do choose to consume legumes, sprouting, soaking, and fermenting will reduce the phytic acid content significantly. In many cases, these processes can almost entirely remove phytic acid and may substantially increase the nutritional value of these foods. In some cases, however, legumes can be quite aggravating to digestion. If you notice bloating or digestive discomfort after eating them, they may be best to avoid while you are going through the healing process.

Beverages

As we all know, water is absolutely the best beverage of all. It's what our body really needs. Women with PCOS often lose weight more easily when they increase their water intake. It's phenomenal what this one simple act can do. A recent study in *The American Journal of Clinical Nutrition* found that when subjects replaced diet soda with water after each meal on a twenty-four-week weight loss program, they lost fourteen percent more weight, and their insulin resistance markers improved by forty-one percent.[11]

If you are wondering how well hydrated you are, you can measure by the color of your urine. If it is lighter, it's a sign you are probably getting enough water. Strong-smelling or dark-colored urine is a sign you need more. That is, unless you are taking B vitamins. Vitamin B1 changes the color of your urine to a fluorescent yellow hue, which is completely normal. Another at-home test you can do to check your hydration is to purchase some chemstrips online. The specific gravity is the measure of how concentrated your urine is. Aim for a specific gravity of less than 1.10. Anything above means that you are moderately dehydrated.

Other healthy beverages include—

- Herbal teas. Spearmint is particularly PCOS friendly, as it lowers androgens.

- Sparkling water. You can pick some up at the grocery store, or you can make your own at home with a Sodastream and some filtered water. You can add lemon, lime, or a few berries to your sparkling water for a delicious healthy treat.

- Green tea. Covered in several sections of this book, green tea has numerous health benefits for women with PCOS, including reducing insulin resistance and combating inflammation.

- Vegetable juices. Juicing at home is an excellent way to add condensed nutrition to your diet. Drink plenty of vegetable juices if you can afford a juicer for home use. The benefits will be enormous!

Coffee

Coffee is something that I personally enjoy, but I have done research into whether it is healthy or harmful. It depends on your individual condition overall; however, it can actually be a healthy part of your diet.

The pros of coffee are that it has clear benefits for your brain function. It can improve your mood, your focus, and your concentration, and according to significant research, it can keep neurodegenerative processes, such as Alzheimer's disease, at bay.[12] It also boosts your metabolism, a clear benefit for women with PCOS. However, if you drink coffee every day, this effect may wear off in time. People who drink coffee have also been found to have a lower incidence of metabolic syndrome and lower triglycerides, presumably due to its effects on insulin resistance.[13] In addition to this, coffee contains antioxidants, which may have numerous benefits for cell health.

The cons of coffee are in part related to its stimulating effects. For those with anxiety, or those who have adrenal hyperactivity and high cortisol levels, it may actually exacerbate and aggravate their condition. It can cause insomnia, so those who already suffer from insomnia should avoid it entirely. It can also be irritating to the gastrointestinal tract, both due to its stimulating nature and to some of its physical composition. It is also not recommended for women who are pregnant or trying to conceive, as there have really been no clearly established safety rules for pregnancy.

That being said, I do think that most women with PCOS can enjoy moderate amounts of coffee (1–2 cups per day), if they tolerate it. It can boost mood, ward off depression, increase exercise results, and improve metabolic health. Each person is unique in their ability to tolerate and metabolize coffee. Some cannot metabolize caffeine, and the effects will be magnified in these individuals. I recommend that women with PCOS take their coffee black. This may be a stretch; however, you'll find that after a short period of time, you will not miss the sugar or cream.

Foods to Avoid

Now we are going to look at foods that can trigger symptoms in those suffering from PCOS. I recommend avoiding the foods listed in this section to reduce your symptoms as you work to reverse your PCOS. I just want to make a note here about nutritional restriction. In most cases, the strict avoidance of the foods on this list is not necessary, or even healthy. Although it is helpful to avoid certain foods in general, if you eat something on the avoid list occasionally, it will not have much of a negative impact. It's important not to let nutrition be a stressor for you and to know that perfection isn't required to make changes that will transform your health. There are some exceptions: For those wanting to lose weight, following these guidelines more closely will definitely result in more success. For those who have intolerances, or autoimmune diseases that are aggravated by specific food triggers, you probably already know that more compliance is needed to support your health.

My goal is not for you to look at foods as either good or bad, but rather to learn to make the best choices on a daily basis. These choices often come naturally when you are armed with information on nutrition, and you'll feel at your best when you focus on eating real, whole foods.

Sugar

This is the number one thing that should be avoided if you have PCOS. As we know, many foods contain natural sugar, and we'll need to watch that also since as women with PCOS we are far more sensitive to all types of sugar, both natural and added. However, it's the added sugars that are particularly harmful, because they tend to be more dense and without nutrients like fiber, vitamins, and minerals.

I often recommend avoiding all types of sugar, whether it's fructose or glucose. Sugar in the form of glucose directly increases insulin, and women with PCOS have shown intense inflammatory responses to a dose of sugar almost immediately after ingestion.[14] Women without PCOS don't have this same inflammatory response. As such, we need to be much more careful about our sugar consumption than others do.

Fructose, however, is a different animal. Sucrose—what we typically call "table sugar"—is about half fructose and half glucose. Glucose can be absorbed and metabolized by all of the different cells in the body through the action of insulin. Fructose, however, is different: It is primarily absorbed by the liver without the help of insulin. As a result, fructose doesn't raise the blood sugar or insulin level much after it is consumed. Instead, the liver takes it up and stores it into an energy form known as glycogen, which is basically a storage tank of sugar within the liver. When a small amount of fructose is consumed, such as in a small serving of fruit, the body can handle this easily.

When we fast, when we sleep, for example, the body will use up the glycogen in the liver for fuel. The same thing happens after we exercise, because exercising also requires the burning of the glycogen, which is stored. This is why having some starchy carbohydrate is a good idea after exercise: It refills the tank of glycogen that has been depleted.

It's a totally different matter, however, when a large amount of fructose is consumed, particularly when the glycogen tank is already full (which it is, most of the time). The excess fructose has nowhere to go and must be converted into fat, much of which deposits right in the liver. This action is linked to causing nonalcoholic fatty liver disease (NAFLD), which is a common PCOS-related condition.

Eating too much fructose has also been associated with increased abdominal fat deposition, cardiovascular disease, and insulin resistance. For more information about this condition, which is common in women with PCOS, please see Appendix C.

Fructose also decreases circulating insulin and leptin levels when it enters your system and increases ghrelin levels.[15] Because leptin and insulin decrease appetite and ghrelin increases appetite, it's thought that this may be why fructose has been linked to weight gain.

Sugar and the Microbiome
Sugar also disrupts the bacterial balance within our small intestines, shifting the millions of microorganisms that reside there, known as the microbiome, and changing the very type of species that live there. Eating a lot of sugar, or a standard Western diet, can shift the microbiome toward one that is associated with obesity and insulin resistance.[16]

The microbes that live in our gut can either help us have good metabolic health, or they can hinder us and contribute to insulin resistance, obesity, and inflammation.

Sugar feeds the wrong types of bacteria, causing them to flourish and overgrow, leaving little room for the friendly bacteria that are linked to good metabolic health.

There are two prominent intestinal bacterial species, known as the fermicutes and bacteriodes. When these species are in good equilibrium, our metabolism is healthy, but when the ratio of these is poor in the intestine, the person will actually gain weight. Transplantation of bacteria from insulin-resistant medically "obese" donors into a recipient can actually cause weight gain.[17] It's thought that differences in the microbiome even play a large role in our resting metabolic rate and how many calories we burn while asleep. Over time, we will learn more, but it's clear that the microbiome plays a huge role in our metabolic health, inflammation, and insulin resistance.

Non-Sugar Sweeteners: Natural and Artificial

When it comes to sweeteners, I generally ask my patients to avoid even natural sweeteners for a period of thirty days. This is to reduce their desire for sweet and to turn off the areas of the brain that are asking them to eat sugar. Artificial sweeteners may be able to disrupt the insulin pathways, creating a similar response to sugar in the brain. In addition, some studies have even found that artificial sweeteners may increase hunger, cravings, and/or food intake.[18] I recommend that you avoid these entirely.

Become a Sugar Detective

In this section, I've included a list of sugars to avoid. Note that sugars are often hidden skillfully under a variety of names on a label. You'll want to become familiar with these so you can detect them before buying a food. Being sugar savvy will help you on your journey toward better health.

These sugars in the following list are names you may recognize from packaging. Keep an eye out for them, as these are all different forms of sugar:

- Glucose
- Dextrose
- Lactose
- Maltose
- Sucrose
- Galactose
- Saccharose
- Corn syrup
- Brown rice syrup

Natural Sugars

Generally, it's also best to avoid natural sugars, but they can be enjoyed occasionally as part of a treat. Of the natural sugars listed here, blackstrap molasses offers a good nutritional punch, as it includes iron, calcium, magnesium, manganese, antioxidants, and vitamin B6. Date sugar is another good choice, as it is the natural sugar richest in antioxidants and is quite sweet, so less can be used.

- Date sugar
- Blackstrap molasses
- Maple syrup
- Honey (contains forty percent fructose, but it contains beneficial antioxidants)

High-Fructose "Natural" Sugars

These are not recommended for women with PCOS as a general rule. Concentrated fructose, as mentioned earlier, is metabolized through the liver, can raise triglycerides, and contributes to fatty liver. It is also associated with weight gain. Try to avoid the following for that reason:

- Fructose
- Agave nectar
- Coconut sugar (contains seventy percent sucrose, half of which is fructose)

Natural Non-Caloric Sweeteners

Stevia is the leaf of a plant known as *Stevia rebaudiana*. Stevia has an intensely sweet taste, and so very little of it is required to sweeten. Overall, it's very likely to be safe when consumed occasionally and in small amounts. One caution with stevia is that it has been linked to infertility in animal studies, so women who are trying to conceive should avoid it. If stevia is used, natural green leaf stevia is the best type.

Sugar Alcohols

These are forms of sugar that are slightly different in structure, having an extra oxygen and hydrogen atom attached. This puts them into the category of a sugar alcohol. These do occur naturally in fruits but only in small quantities. The sugar alcohols are less sweet than sugar, have fewer calories than sugar, and have less of an effect in raising blood glucose. Unfortunately, many people react with digestive symptoms, such as bloating, gas, and diarrhea, upon eating sugar alcohols. This is because they are poorly absorbed and travel down to the colon and act as substrate for certain types of bacteria in the gut. In some individuals, this can seriously aggravate intestinal health. As such, they are generally best to avoid; however, of the list provided, erythrytol is the best choice, as it is absorbed almost completely in the small intestine, avoiding passage to the colon and fermentation by microbes:

- Xylitol
- Erythrytol
- Sorbitol

Artificial Sweeteners

Artificial sweeteners should be avoided. They have been linked to insulin resistance and can alter the human microbiome. Most of all, my main concern with them is that there is evidence suggesting that certain artificial sweeteners may be linked to cancer. Until more safety information is available, it is definitely best to avoid these altogether and choose from the many other options for the occasional consumption of sweetener. These sweeteners include—

- Aspartame
- Sucralose
- Saccharin
- Acesulfame-K

Dairy

The dairy industry has told us repeatedly that dairy is a health food and is actually required in order to be healthy. This is not the case at all. Now, some people do feel very well with quality dairy products. However, the reality is that for PCOS, dairy is something that should be avoided.

When you think about dairy, what is its purpose? Milk is a food that is made to nourish a baby animal before it can consume nutrients through other food sources. As such, it is biologically engineered to stimulate and support the rapid growth of a young animal. It is nutrient dense and made to provide a large amount of everything needed to support tissue growth, all within a very small volume. This is great for a baby animal with a relatively small stomach that is growing at a very rapid pace.

However, does this seem like something we should be having if we are insulin resistant and are already metabolic conservers? Absolutely not! As we saw when we went through the insulin index, dairy products, even fermented ones, such as yogurt, are some of the most insulinemic foods out there. In fact, on the insulin index, yogurt rates as high as white bread!

In particular, amino acids, the building blocks of protein, especially the branched chain variety (valine, isoleucine, and leucine), can cause a spike of insulin that is quite significant. Dairy contains these amino acids. So, for women with PCOS, it wreaks havoc with insulin levels in a similar manner as white bread. In addition to the specific amino acids in dairy that cause our insulin levels to spike, dairy also contains several other compounds that are concerning for metabolic health. For a baby animal, these compounds have an important and useful function. In an adult, they may present issues depending on your metabolic health status. For example, dairy contains—

- Insulin
- Leptin
- Insulin-like growth factors
- Various forms of estrogen, including—
    - Estrone
    - Estriol
    - 17-alpha estradiol
    - 17-beta estradiol
- Progesterone
- Testosterone
- Cortisol

Cow's milk contains considerable amounts of female sex hormones in particular. These may compound the already existing hormonal imbalances in PCOS. In addition, since women with PCOS are more at risk for endometrial cancer, the consumption of additional estrogen in dairy would be concerning, given its link to cancer.

In modern dairy production, cows are milked hundreds of times per year and are pregnant for much of that time. Toward the end of pregnancy, the amount of female sex hormones in the milk is quite high. This could also be a very important factor to consider for mothers of daughters with PCOS, since seventy-five percent of children consume dairy daily. The amount of estrogen that girls at risk for PCOS are consuming in the pubertal period could have unknown health outcomes years from now. Studies have already linked hormonally positive cancers of the breast and prostate to dairy consumption, so there just isn't any good reason to be consuming this food. Of course, dairy produced in a more natural way, or purchased from a farm where more natural methods are practiced, would contain much lower levels of hormones.

Overall, such a nutrient-dense, made-to-build-tissue food may work wonderfully in the calf's body, for which it was designed. However, for an adult woman who has the tendency to deposit abdominal fat, this is the exact opposite of what we should be eating. The leptin in milk also contributes further to the leptin resistance that many women with PCOS are fighting against. IGF-1 and IGF-2 are also growth-promoting factors. As such, we do not need to be directly consuming these either.

Then we come to the steroid hormones, namely the estrogen, testosterone, progesterone, and cortisol that are present in milk. In a system that is already prone to hormonal flatline, adding more to that mix will only further confuse our receptors, our hypothalamus, and our ovaries. Our goal is to restore the normal signaling environment of the hormones, one that is primarily disrupted in PCOS. Dairy products only serve to further confuse our hormonal systems, and for that reason, I ask most women with PCOS to avoid them entirely.

Table 9-4: Reported Endocrine Factors Found in Bovine Colostrum and Milk

ENDOCRINE FACTOR	COLOSTRUM	MILK	SOURCE
IGF-1	1–3 µg/mL	10–50 ng/mL	Malven et al. (1987)
IGF-2	1.8 µg/mL	1–20 ng/mL	Vega et al. (1991)
IGFBPs	~3 µg/mL	~2 µg/mL	Puvogel et al. (2005)
EGF (likely betacellulin)	3 ng/mL	1.5 ng/mL	Iacopetta et al. (1992); Xiao et al. (2002)
Betacellulin	2.3 ng/mL	~2 ng/mL	Bastian et al. (2001)
TGF α	2.2–7.2 µg/mL	0–8.4 µg/mL	
TGF-β2	74 ng/mL; act: 150–1150 ng/mL		Pakkanen (1998)
TGF-β2 1&2	?	8 ng/mL	Cox and Burk (1991)
FGF (acidic)	?	~6 ng/mL	Rogers et al. (1995)
FGF (basic)	?	~20 ng/mL	Rogers et al. (1995)
Insulin	6–37 ng/mL	4–7 ng/mL	Malven et al. (1987)
Prolactin	500–800 ng/mL	6–8 ng/mL	KacsÓh et al. (1991)
Leptin	13.9 ng/mL	6.1 ng/mL	Pinotti and Rosi (2006)

Table 9-5: Insulin-Like Growth Factors Binding Proteins

ENDOCRINE LIGAND	COLOSTRUM	MILK	COMMERCIAL MILK[B]	SOURCE
Estrone	2000–4000	9.2–118[c]	8–20[c]	Malekinejad et al. (2006); Janowski et al. (2002); Pope and Roy (1953)
17 α Estradiol	?	7–47[d]	nd[c]	Malekinejad et al. (2006)
17 β Estradiol	1500–2000[d] 1000[f]	6–221[c]	10–20[c]	Malekinejad et al. (2006); Janowski et al. (2002); Pope and Roy (1953)
Estriol	?	nd[c]	nd[c]	Malekinejad et al. (2006)
Progesterone	?	11,300[c]	2,100–11,000[c]	Fritsche and Steinhart (1999)
Testosterone	?	50–150[c]	10[ef]	Fritsche and Steinhart (1999)
Cortisol	1,590–4,400[d]	350[d]	710[d]	Butler and Des Bordes (1980); Shutt and Fell (1985)

Source: Blum and Baumrucker, 2008; Pape-Zambito, Roberts, and Kensinger, 2010

I am not totally against dairy as a general rule, and it is true that quality, grass-fed dairy products can provide good nutrition for some individuals. However, in the typical woman with PCOS, they are arguably one of the most important foods to avoid.

My patients often ask me how they can get their calcium if they do not consume dairy. The first thing to note is that consuming large amounts of calcium, as we have been advised by government agencies, does not necessarily correlate with reduced fracture risk. The World Health Organization has reduced its recommendations for the consumption of calcium in favor of exercise (which has proven to benefit bone density), maintaining good vitamin D levels, and increasing the consumption of fruits and vegetables.

Protein can actually increase the excretion of calcium,[19] so we must look at calcium intake as a function of the overall diet you are following. If you are consuming calcium with animal protein, such as cow's milk, the absorption is far less than what you might think. If you are eating a healthy diet, avoiding processed foods, consuming a large variety of calcium-rich, healthy, leafy green vegetables, and getting regular exercise, you should easily reach the amount of calcium recommended. Beware of calcium supplements, particularly those of lower quality. Though the label may read a large amount of calcium, only a small amount is actually absorbed by the body.

Table 9-6: Calcium-Rich Foods

FOOD	SERVING SIZE	CALCIUM/ STANDARD SERVING	CALCIUM ABSORBED/ SERVING[2]	AMOUNT NEEDED TO ABSORB ~100 mg Ca
		mg	mg	
2% milk	1 cup	297	95	1 cup
Cheddar cheese	1 oz	204	66	1–½ oz
Sesame seeds, unhulled	1 oz	280	58	1–¾ oz
Kale, frozen	½ cup	90	53	1 cup
Turnip greens, frozen	½ cup	99	51	1 cup
Mustard greens, frozen	½ cup	76	44	1–⅛ oz
Chinese cabbage, bok choy, boiled	½ cup	79	43	1–⅛ oz
White beans, cooked	1 cup	161	35	2–¾ oz
Broccoli, frozen	½ cup	47	29	1–⅔ oz
Brussels sprouts, boiled	½ cup	28	18	2–¾ oz
Spinach, boiled	½ cup	122	6	8 cups

In the Harvard Nurses' Health Study, which followed more than 70,000 women for more than twelve years, it was found that consuming dairy products had no effect on the fracture risk in these women.[20] If after increasing your consumption of green leafy vegetables you feel you are still deficient in reaching your requirements for calcium, it's much better to choose a quality calcium supplement to achieve your daily needs. Until recently, the recommended daily amount of calcium for women of reproductive age has been approximately 1,000 mg. However, several health agencies have recently made changes to their recommendations on calcium requirements. The World Health Organization now recommends 500 mg per day, and Dr. Walter Willett, chair of the Department of Nutrition at the Harvard T. H. Chan School of

Public Health, agrees. He states that high-dose calcium doesn't provide any benefits and that between 500 and 700 mg per day should suffice.

When it comes to supplementation, there are differences between the forms of calcium. Many inexpensive forms of calcium, such as calcium carbonate, do not have the same ability to slow the breakdown process of bone. In fact, studies have found that better forms of calcium, such as calcium citrate, may have increased benefits in slowing bone breakdown by as much as thirty percent. Other forms, which also have good absorption, include calcium malate and calcium hydroxy-apatite. However, as hydroxyapatite is sourced from an animal (usually cows), the brand must be chosen carefully.

Some foods are also fortified with calcium. Dairy alternatives abound these days and there are many to choose from. The options include—

- Almond milk
- Coconut milk
- Rice milk
- Cashew milk
- Quinoa milk
- Soy milk

I do not recommend that women with PCOS consume soy milk, for reasons I'll explain later. My favorites of the milks listed for women with PCOS are almond milk, cashew milk, and coconut milk. Each has a slightly different profile, with almond milk generally being the lowest in calories. Cashew milk and coconut milk offer a higher healthy fat profile and are more filling. Rice milk is higher in carbohydrates and therefore not the best option.

Many boxed-milk alternatives contain carrageenan, which can irritate the intestines for some individuals. There are now organic brands that are free of this additive, so read your labels. Even better: You may want to try making your own nut milks. It's very easy with a blender.

Gluten

Gluten, which is found in wheat, spelt, rye, and barley, is a food I recommend that women with PCOS avoid, for the most part, though this may vary from woman to woman. Gluten is made up of gliadin and glutenin. The gliadin is the problematic part for most individuals. In people with celiac disease, reactions to gluten can be severe, damaging the intestines and causing severe destruction of the intestinal cells.

However, only one percent of the population has celiac disease, so how does that apply to you?

First, gluten can be an inflammatory food. It creates leaky gut and triggers immune reactions in many people. A growing body of evidence suggests that a large percentage of people who do not have celiac disease are sensitive to gluten, primarily because of these inflammatory effects. Some people may have antibodies to gluten in their stool or blood, yet they do not have celiac disease. Those who are sensitive secrete increased amounts of a protein known as zonulin in their intestines after consuming gluten. This protein causes the intestinal barrier to leak, which can create a host of negative effects for intestinal health. Around forty percent of people carry the genes for celiac disease, predisposing them to sensitivities to gluten, even though they may never develop full-blown celiac disease. Now, thankfully out of the realm of being considered an imaginary syndrome, non-celiac gluten sensitivity has been confirmed as a real condition with increased intestinal permeability responses to gluten ingestion, without the autoimmunity of celiac disease.[21]

As women with PCOS have an excessive amount of inflammation, this is problematic. I've found that many women with PCOS feel much better without gluten as part of their diet. The only real way to know if you are sensitive to gluten is to eliminate it from your diet for a month. If you feel better, don't eat it! That being said, it is not necessary for the vast majority of women with PCOS to avoid gluten to the degree that someone with celiac disease would.

It's also interesting to note that gluten can have negative effects on anyone, even if they are not particularly sensitive to it. It causes permeability of the gut lining, allowing products from the intestine to activate inflammatory responses, and has been linked to irritable bowel syndrome.[22]

One of the best reasons to avoid gluten is that it increases leptin resistance. A recent study showed a fifty percent increase in leptin resistance after cells were exposed to gluten.[23] Leptin resistance increases hunger, causing us to eat more. This may be why wheat is addictive, in a similar way sugar is. Gluten also contains small peptides called exorphins, with opioid-like properties that some researchers believe play a role in its addictiveness.

Grains

When it comes to grains in general, there may be good reason to minimize their consumption. Many grains contain similarly irritating, inflammatory substances such as gliadin. Grains, such as corn, are one of the more common allergens, and the vast majority are genetically modified.

Grains also contain phytates. Phytates have received mixed reviews, so I'd like to take a closer look with you. Phytates are found in plant seeds (grains) and have been referred to as "anti-nutrients." Phytates are also found in legumes and certain nuts, which I'll discuss in the next section. The amount of phytates in foods is variable as well.

The main argument against phytates is that they decrease the absorption of different minerals, including iron, zinc, and calcium. This effect is only present directly after eating the food itself and doesn't last for long periods of time. So, as you can see, phytates are something that you wouldn't want to be consuming with every meal, or you could potentially develop nutritional deficiencies over time. In addition, if you are consuming a variety of foods with phytates, you increase this effect exponentially. Therefore, I would suggest that it's best to be selective with your phytates: mostly nuts and some legumes, if you are able to tolerate them.

Phytates are not all bad. They do have antioxidant and anti-cancer properties. As such, we have to look at them as something to balance in our diet rather than be afraid of. Although grains, such as buckwheat, contain inositols, a compound we know is quite beneficial for women with PCOS, the inositol must be cleaved from the phytates within to be accessed. As such, I do not recommend that women obtain their inositols from grains, because to get the recommended amount, a large quantity would have to be consumed, and this could disrupt the absorption of other minerals from the diet.

Rice may be an exception and is most likely one of the best-tolerated grains, because it tends to have little allergenic potential. That being said, its high insulin index means that it should be used in small quantities only. In addition, although brown rice has been long recommended as the healthier rice, it contains higher amounts of phytic acid, which, for reasons stated earlier, may negate some of its benefits. The occasional consumption of small amounts of steel cut oats or quinoa would also be an exception for those who are not sensitive to these, but this should be done within the following insulin index guidelines.

The Ideal Macronutrient Structure for Your Meals

Before calculating the insulin counts of your meals, the first step is learning to structure the components on your plate—protein, vegetables, carbohydrates, and fat. Start with lean protein. The portion should be about the size of the palm of your hand. Depending on the protein you choose and your recommended insulin count, which we will address next, you may be able to have more or less. You'll get a lot more portion-wise from choosing poultry or fish when compared to beef. Half of your plate should be comprised of vegetables. Add a serving of healthy fats (around one tablespoon of a healthy oil or one serving of avocado or nuts).

Finally, add a small serving of carbohydrates. Choose from the most nutritionally dense and least inflammatory carbohydrates first, like berries, sweet potatoes, and squash. Yes, that's right, fruits are carbohydrates! You can occasionally have quinoa or white or brown rice if your body tolerates it. Bread is not recommended, particularly for those who want to lose weight, as it is typically made of processed grains and almost always contains gluten. There are, however, some gluten- and grain-free homemade breads high in healthy fats and proteins that are an exception.

Your Ideal Insulin Count

Now that you've got an idea of how to structure your plate, let's talk about insulin counting. The insulin count that is best for you depends on a few different things, including your level of insulin resistance, your desire to achieve weight loss, and your personal response to different levels of carbohydrate restriction. Once you are used to the process of insulin counting, my hope is that you will be able to estimate your most optimal meal structure without measuring or calculating. At first, you may want to invest in a small kitchen scale and some measuring cups to get familiar with the recommended portions, particularly if weight loss is your goal.

Insulin counting is very easy: You simply add up the count of each food or ingredient in your meal. Adjust the count for the quantity that you consume. So, if you have double the quantity listed of a food, just double the insulin count. As insulin indices have been measured for certain foods, there are likely many foods you would like to enjoy that are not included. In this case, just substitute the insulin count of the most similar food when it comes to carbohydrate or protein content. In time, the list will grow and many more foods will be included.

Insulin Count Guidelines

As a general rule, for women who are insulin resistant, carry extra weight around the abdomen, or who want to lose a significant amount of weight, aiming for an insulin count of between fifty and sixty per meal is often optimal. Some women may do even better under fifty, but this should be supervised by a health-care practitioner.

Table 9-7: Foods and Insulin Counts for Women with Significant Insulin Resistance

SAMPLE CHOICE	INSULIN COUNT
Four ounces of roast chicken breast	17
Two cups of green vegetables	5
One half of an avocado	4
One half of a medium sweet potato (76 g)	23
Total	49

SAMPLE CHOICE	INSULIN COUNT
Four ounces of white fish	15
Two cups of mashed cauliflower	12
One tablespoon of extra virgin olive oil	2
One cup of leafy green salad with lemon juice	0
One apple	15
Total	44

For women who are of average weight and mildly insulin resistant, start with an insulin count of approximately fifty-five to sixty-five per meal.

Table 9-8: Additional Foods and Insulin Counts

SAMPLE CHOICE	INSULIN COUNT
Four ounces of roast chicken breast	17
Two cups of cooked broccoli	5
Half an avocado	4
Half a cup of rice	24
Total	50

For women with PCOS who are underweight, very lean, athletic, and not insulin-resistant, aim for an insulin count between sixty-five and ninety, as needed to support energy levels. You'll soon learn what feels best.

Table 9-9: Additional Foods and Insulin Counts for Lean PCOS—Non-Insulin Resistant

SAMPLE CHOICE	INSULIN COUNT
Six ounces roast chicken breast	26
Two cups of cooked cauliflower	12
Half an avocado	4
Half a cup of rice	24
One peach	10
Total	76

Adequate insulin is needed to support leptin levels in the brain. This is why the very low-carb approach is often unsuccessful in women with PCOS who are underweight, very lean, and non-insulin resistant. This is particularly true for those women who have difficulty gaining weight. Typical recommended eating plans for PCOS can actually make matters worse in this situation. In these cases, there is a predisposition to low leptin, and going too low on the insulin count can shock the hypothalamus and interfere with ovulation. I usually recommend adding extra protein for women such as this. As you'll see in the next table, additional protein is included as well as ensuring that at least thirty-five points are achieved through carbohydrates at each meal.

Table 9-10: Sample Foods and Insulin Counts for Very Lean or Athletic Women with PCOS

SAMPLE CHOICE	INSULIN COUNT
175 grams roast chicken breast	25.5
Two cups of cooked cauliflower	20
One half of an avocado	4
1 serving baked sweet potato fries	37
Dessert: One peach	9
Total	95.5

Some very athletic women will need many more calories than this to support their activity level, so follow the same general structure for your meal and increase the amount of each food, but try to keep the composition approximately the same. Additional mini-meals and snacks should also be added as needed for very active women.

Again, this does not have to be exact, particularly in those who don't need or want to lose weight, but it serves as a general guideline that can be followed. Over time, you'll learn how to combine your foods for optimal insulin responses in your body—and your insulin sensitivity will gradually increase. In addition, there are always exceptions, and some of you may feel best at a higher or lower insulin count than your category indicates. I would tell you to listen to your body and adjust to what feels right for you!

For those who want to lose significant weight, it may be beneficial to determine your ideal intake with a nutritional practitioner, such as a naturopathic doctor, dietician, or nutritionist, as you'll be able to get the personalized guidance you need along your journey.

Following are some guidelines for you as you plan your meals and snacks. I have included some recommended diets, along with sample recipes, for you in Appendix D. Also, please visit my page at http://www.drfionand.com/insulincount for calculators to help you with determining and tracking your insulin count.

Sample PCOS Meal Plans
Breakfast

According to research, a breakfast high in healthy fats is associated with metabolic benefits for the rest of the day.[24] Because fats are low on the insulin index, you may find that a lower insulin count of 35–45 for breakfast may be beneficial, particularly if you are insulin resistant. As always, it's important to listen to your body and do what feels best for you. Smoothies are a great option, as they are fast, easy, and nutritious. I always recommend the following format:

- 25 grams of protein powder (vegan or collagen)
- 1 cup of vegetables (choose from romaine, kale, dandelion, collards, spinach, or another green)
- Choice of 2 cups frozen berries, ½ orange, 1 peach, or ½ apple
- 1–½ cups of unsweetened almond or coconut milk
- Choice of ¼ avocado, 1 tablespoon of coconut oil, or 2 tablespoons of nut butter
- 1 tablespoon of chia seeds
- Raw cacao or coconut (for extra flavor)

I'd like for you to think outside the box. Most women with PCOS can't handle high carbohydrate loads very well, and most of our traditional breakfasts are carbohydrate based, so we need to think outside of traditional Western-style breakfasts and make choices that are healthy for us. I recommend having a serving of vegetables with each and every meal, including breakfast.

Eggs are a popular breakfast food, and to add vegetables, we can enjoy omelets with onions, peppers, mushrooms, and spinach for breakfast. Some other breakfast choices include—

- Two eggs, poached or over easy with stir-fried mushrooms and cabbage as a side dish (Add some sea salt and apple cider vinegar to the vegetables as you cook them for extra flavor.)
- Root veggie hash (Sauteé sweet potatoes, cabbage, and chicken with sea salt. Serve with a poached egg.)
- All-natural, organic breakfast sausage with veggies on the side
- Low-carb, high-protein "muffins" made with almond flour (You can make these ahead of time and freeze them. See recipe for "Protein-Packed Apple Cinnamon Muffins" in Appendix D.)
- Egg muffins to go (See recipe for "Egg Muffins with Prosciutto" in Appendix D.)

Lunches and Dinners

As a general rule, you'll want to portion your meals as already outlined. This should, as a general rule, produce a good insulin count. Choose a protein source approximately the size and thickness of the palm of your hand. Fill the rest of your plate with vegetables. Add a healthy fat source, such as avocado; some healthy oil, such as coconut oil, avocado oil, or extra virgin olive oil; or two tablespoons of nuts or seeds. Also, stop eating altogether after dinnertime. If you are hungry, have a glass of herbal tea, sparkling water with lemon, or even better, meditate, exercise, or read. This will produce a time of intermittent fasting which many report helps with weight loss.

Quick Healthy Solutions

Sometimes you won't have time to make an elaborate meal. As such, you can make these quick meals in a matter of minutes that will be full of nutrition and will keep your blood sugar stable:

- Hard-boiled eggs with broccoli florets, a small handful of nuts, and an apple
- Canned wild Alaska salmon with mixed organic greens and a handful of blueberries
- Zucchini noodles with turkey meat sauce (Consider purchasing a spiralizer to make quick veggie noodles.)
- Taco salad of romaine lettuce topped with ground turkey and chili seasoning, avocados, tomatoes, and bell peppers
- Egg scramble with veggies and coconut oil
- Broiled salmon with mashed turnips on the side

- Pan-fried fish with salad
- Chili (either vegetarian or omnivorous)
- Anything made in the crockpot with protein, vegetables, and a small amount of root vegetables, like sweet potato or squash

See Appendix D for a week's meal plan with recipes.

Snacking
Women with Mild to Significant Insulin Resistance
When it comes to snacking, it is always good to preplan your snacks and to avoid grazing outside of your snacking times. One morning and one afternoon snack with an insulin count of less than fifteen is ideal. Some women who are severely insulin resistant actually do far better avoiding snacking between meals, as this allows insulin levels to drop when not eating. Some examples include—

- One ounce of nuts (a closed handful) and half a piece of fruit
- Carrot sticks or romaine lettuce leaves dipped in guacamole
- Chia pudding
- Almond flour muffin
- Broccoli slaw with homemade mayo
- Slivered almonds with blueberries in coconut milk
- Two boiled eggs

Women Who Are Non-Insulin Resistant, Athletic, or Underweight
It's always best to preplan your snacks. However, if you feel hungry, you may add additional snacks as needed. One morning and one afternoon snack with an insulin count of around twenty is a good idea. Some examples of healthy snacks include—

- One apple and a handful of nuts
- A shake with twenty grams of protein and berries
- Slivered almonds with blueberries in coconut milk
- Almond flour muffins
- Chia pudding
- Two boiled eggs and carrot sticks
- Cucumber slices with guacamole
- A handful of grapes with two macadamia nuts

Post-Workout Snacks

All women with PCOS should have a snack within fifteen to twenty minutes of working out. This snack should be low in fat and contain carbohydrates and protein. An insulin count of around twenty to thirty is best. Some good examples include—

- A shake (twenty grams of protein) with half of a banana
- An egg-white omelet with a few sweet potato chunks
- One quarter of a cold, baked sweet potato with tuna

Intermittent Fasting

For women who are significantly insulin resistant and who find it very challenging to lose weight around the abdomen despite making dietary changes and exercising, intermittent fasting can help break this pattern. The most basic type of intermittent fasting involves fasting after dinner for a fourteen-hour span. In those who are severely insulin resistant, insulin levels can remain very high, and fasting allows the insulin levels to drop. Intermittent fasting is often an easy way to address the plateaus of weight loss resistance. Part of insulin's action is to inhibit the breakdown of fat, but when levels are continuously high, as they are in insulin resistant people, the cells remain in storage mode. Each time we eat, our insulin levels rise again. Fasting gives the metabolic system a break, and it has no choice but to release stored fat. Intermittent fasting can range from hours to days. Please see the resources section or visit my website for more information.

Overall, this nutrition plan offers a lot of flexibility, as most types of healthy, whole foods can be included. Insulin counting gives you a method to manage the impact that foods are having on your PCOS by managing the single most aggravating nutritional factor to the condition: foods that spike insulin levels. When you eat well-structured meals as a habit, you'll feel better. It also helps prevent disease and heals your metabolism. And when you choose whole, real, clean foods, you'll be safeguarding not only your health but that of future generations as well. Two tablespoons of vinegar before meals and at bedtime may improve insulin sensitivity for those who are insulin resistant. Raw apple cider vinegar is a popular choice because it also contains fiber as a pectin.

This program is not meant to be a restrictive diet plan, but rather a new way of viewing food and nutrition for the betterment of your overall health. I hope that you'll be able to take this information and use it as a stepping-stone to learning the most optimal way of eating for your unique expression of PCOS.

Appendix A
PCOS AND FERTILITY

Even miracles take a little time.
—FAIRY GODMOTHER

Thirty-six-year-old Maria had been married for three years. Maria was a medium-framed woman with brown hair and green eyes who had the tendency to carry a little extra weight around her middle. As soon as she met her husband, they decided to begin their family. Unfortunately, Maria's PCOS had something else in mind. Maria's periods had never been very regular, and her cycles ranged from thirty-three to forty-three days. Maria also suffered from some of the other characteristics of PCOS. Last year, she had undergone a multitude of laser sessions to remove unwanted facial hair. Her joints ached on a daily basis, and she had various allergies. Maria's ultrasounds showed the classic string-of-pearls appearance. Maria had Type 1 classic PCOS. Her factors included high androgens, ovulatory dysfunction, insulin resistance, and inflammation.

After trying to conceive for a whole year, not only was Maria still not pregnant, it also seemed more and more likely that she wasn't ovulating very often at all. Her friends all seemed to become pregnant within a month or two, which only made matters worse. Every pregnancy announcement felt like a blow to the chest.

Concerned, Maria began tracking her cycle days carefully on a calendar, taking her temperature faithfully each morning and plotting it precisely on a graph. Her temperature line was a long jagged pattern and didn't look like the beautiful two-sectioned charts that she would pore over during her late-night Internet searches. Frustrated, Maria moved on to the expensive ovulation sticks from the drugstore. Stick after stick was used, and nothing made sense: They seemed to constantly be negative, just like her pregnancy tests. In fact, it seemed like all she ever saw was one solid line and a second fainter line, instead of the strong positive line shown on the package. Her frustration grew.

Maria, at her breaking point, visited a local fertility clinic, where she endured several cycles of medication and artificial insemination treatments. These, too, proved unsuccessful. PCOS had wreaked havoc on Maria's hormones, skin, and body: She was determined that this disorder would not also threaten her ability to have children.

PCOS and Infertility

Just like Maria, many women with PCOS have difficulty conceiving. PCOS is the cause of more than seventy-five percent of cases of anovulatory infertility and is a leading cause of infertility in general. Although many women with PCOS do not have any difficulty becoming pregnant, it is definitely one of the most challenging and stressful results of the disorder.

The reason that women with PCOS have trouble conceiving lies in three main concerns:

1. Ovulatory difficulty

2. Hormonal imbalance

3. Increased miscarriage risk

Since one of the three main criteria for PCOS includes delayed ovulation or lack of ovulation, it's quite easy to see why fertility would be affected in many women: Not knowing when you are ovulating is a definite hurdle on the road to becoming pregnant. To make things even more challenging, ovulation prediction kits are often completely inaccurate in women with PCOS. The hormonal marker that is detected with ovulation prediction kits (OPK) is the luteinizing hormone (LH). The control strip of an OPK turns a solid color. The second line measures LH. When LH surges, the second line should turn as dark as the first line. A second line that is lighter than the first is not considered to be a true positive (Figure A-1). In PCOS, LH is often high at unusual times of the cycle. As a result, there can be false positives. OPKs may never register truly positive for women with significant female hormone imbalance and irregular ovulation. This just adds to the massive stress that goes along with trying to conceive.

In addition to not being able to use the most convenient at-home method to detect ovulation, many women like Maria may go several months without ovulating at all. In such cases, there may be little way to know when the most fertile time is coming. Women in these groups have to try to conceive without knowing when is the best time to get pregnant. As such, it's pretty clear why it's no easy to task to make a baby when you have PCOS. Another factor is the egg quality isn't quite what it should be in women with PCOS, as the abundance of testosterone, insulin, and anti-Mullerian hormone alters the structure and function of the follicle.

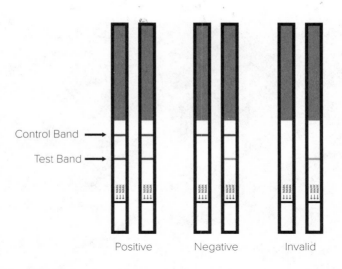

Figure A-1: Hormonal Markers and Ovulation Prediction Kits

Cervical Mucus in PCOS

When it comes to ovulation detection in PCOS, it's not all bad news. One way that women with PCOS may be able to detect their fertile time is through the observation of the cervical mucus. After the menstrual period, a follicle should grow in preparation for ovulation and a dominant follicle will be selected. As the follicle grows, it produces increasing amounts of estrogen. Estrogen stimulates the cells of the cervix to produce a special type of mucus, known as "fertile mucus." This mucus is very similar in texture to that of an egg white. It's slippery and stretchy and can often be noticed when wiping (Figure A-2). At times of the month when fertility is low, the cervical mucus may range in texture from sticky to creamy. Watery cervical mucus is considered to be the second most fertile compared to the egg white texture. So go ahead and try to conceive if you see either of these two types of mucus!

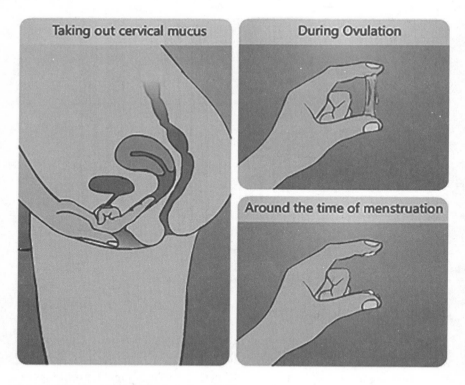

Figure A-2. Testing Cervical Mucus. Copyright Menstrupedia.

A False Peak

When you have PCOS, there are important things you need to know about cervical mucus. When a woman has irregular ovulations, there may be occasions in which the egg begins to grow and release estrogen, and instead of ovulating, it stalls. This initial release of estrogen causes fertile-type cervical mucus to be produced without a corresponding ovulation. This is known as a "false peak." Some women with PCOS even have fertile-type cervical mucus through their entire cycle. As such, we don't know that every production of cervical mucus is a true ovulation, but if you're trying to conceive and you see cervical mucus that is egg white-like in texture, it would definitely be a good idea to try to conceive at that time.

Basal Body Temperature Charting

Basal body temperature (BBT) charting is an excellent way to track cycles in women with PCOS. Through this method, we can determine the length of the follicular phase (the period of time when the egg develops in the ovary prior to ovulation) and the luteal phase (the period of time after ovulation before the menstrual period starts). BBT charting is a very valuable tool for any woman with PCOS who is trying to conceive, so she can identify her patterns and check for luteal-phase defects or low progesterone. The downside of BBT charting is that it is not predictive and generally confirms ovulation *after* it has happened. This is because the basal temperature will rise 0.5–1 degree once ovulation has occurred. In a woman with PCOS, we often see that the first phase of the basal body temperature chart is longer than the typical fourteen days. This is because it takes longer for the eggs to develop under the influence of excess testosterone and LH. Women with PCOS often have a long follicular phase and a short or normal luteal phase. Women in the ovulatory phenotypes, however, may have a normal follicular phase.

You can purchase a basal digital thermometer from any drugstore. The main difference is that most basal thermometers have an additional tenth of a digit and often have a memory that can store your last temperature. However, many women use a regular digital thermometer, which also works very well. Place the thermometer by your bedside and do your best to take your temperature at the same time each morning. Most women use the under-the-tongue method; however, vaginal temperatures are also accurate.

It is important that you take your temperature immediately upon waking, without moving about too much, as this can raise your core temperature. Other things that can decrease the accuracy of your reading are illness, alcohol consumption, insomnia, or taking your temperature at irregular times.

Plot your temperature on a graph. There is a graph for you to print and use on my website at http://drfionand.com/resources/bbtchart. Alternately, there are many wonderful apps available for tracking your basal body temperature—a few are listed in the resources section.

Once you have plotted your temperatures, draw a line connecting the dots on the graph. You should see two distinct patterns within your graph if you have ovulated. Many women with PCOS will not see these two distinct sections, particularly if they have not ovulated. Don't worry if this is the case. BBT charting is really only a tool to learn more about your cycle. If you don't ovulate regularly, you should see improvements in your chart as you undergo treatment, and this can be very exciting!

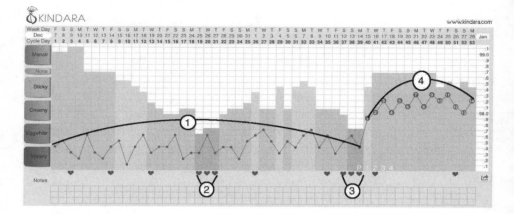

Figure A-3: PCOS Chart

Cervical Position

Fortunately, cervical position seems to be an accurate method of ovulation detection for women with PCOS. The cervix, which is the opening that the sperm must pass through to gain entrance into the uterus, will actually change position as a woman enters her fertile time. Although this method sounds difficult, it is actually quite simple. You'll always want to check your cervical position around the same time each day, as sometimes the cervix will move higher into the vagina at night during sleep. Squatting or propping a foot on the toilet or bathtub can often make it easier to detect the position of the cervix. To check your cervical position, do the following:

1.   Wash your hands and make sure that you don't have any vaginal infections caused by yeast or bacteria.

2.   Gently insert your index or middle finger into your vagina until you feel your cervix. It should feel just like a bump and should be toward the very back part of your vagina.

At the beginning of your cycle, during menstruation, your cervix will feel very firm, like the tip of your nose, and it will be fairly low down and easier to find. The cervix opens during the period, to allow the menstrual fluid to be released. As you approach ovulation, your cervix begins to move up, deeper into the vagina, and may be harder to locate. As you get close to ovulation, the cervix will soften and will open slightly. After ovulation, the cervix closes, becomes firm again, and moves downward. It will remain closed until the period begins.

High-Tech Ways to Identify Ovulation and Cycle Monitoring

If you are attending a fertility clinic or seeing a gynecologist, you may be offered cycle monitoring. Typically, this monitoring involves going into your clinic daily for blood work and ultrasound. If you are menstruating, cycle monitoring will begin on Day 1. For women with PCOS who have irregular menses, cycle monitoring is often done after induction of the period with progesterone.

Bloodwork that is completed on the first day of cycle monitoring often includes follicle-stimulating hormone (FSH), luteinizing hormone (LH), thyroid-stimulating hormone (TSH), estradiol, and progesterone. After Day 1, bloodwork often includes LH, estradiol, and after ovulation, progesterone. To briefly review them, FSH and LH are pituitary hormones. These can indicate the "baseline" of ovarian health. If FSH is high, it can indicate poor egg quality or diminished ovarian reserve. We often see high LH in PCOS. Estradiol should be at a relatively low level on Day 3, and progesterone should be exceptionally low then. Estradiol increases as the follicle grows in preparation for ovulation. Progesterone is released after ovulation occurs.

Typically, cycle monitoring is done early in the morning, as it takes several hours to get the results, and if ovulation is detected, this allows timing of intercourse.

What to Look for in Cycle Monitoring

As your cycle progresses, your ovary will select a dominant follicle that is to be ovulated. As the follicle matures, it produces increasing amounts of estradiol, the main form of estrogen. The average estradiol level from a mature follicle is 200 to 400 pg/ml. As estradiol rises, the pituitary senses this and releases a sharp surge of LH, which triggers ovulation. As the doctor sees that the LH is rising, they may let you know that you are about to ovulate, and that this is a good time to conceive. After ovulation has occurred, the egg will burst from the follicle and begin its journey down the tube. The follicle, still in the ovary but now without its egg, transforms into the corpus luteum. The corpus luteum makes a large amount of progesterone for the rest of the luteal phase, after which time it disintegrates.

A small amount of progesterone is also continuously produced by the adrenal glands. As such, the baseline progesterone levels on cycle day 3 are typically around 1.5 ng/ml or less. Once ovulation has occurred, the progesterone levels rise to 10–18 ng/ml or more by seven days after ovulation (see Figure A-4).

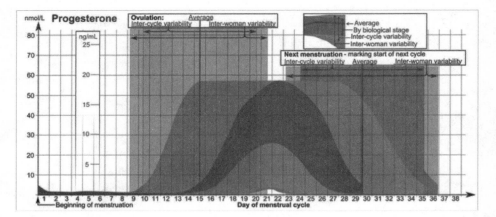

Figure A-4: Progesterone Levels During Menstrual Cycle

Traditional Treatments for Infertility in Women with PCOS

In conventional medicine, treatment for fertility in PCOS typically revolves around what is known as ovulation induction, or "super ovulation." Since lack of ovulation is one of the most important factors impacting fertility in women with PCOS, medications are commonly used to stimulate the ovary to release an egg. However, it's important to know that for women who already ovulate, this type of medication may not increase fertility very much!

Clomiphene

Clomiphene is often the first-line intervention used to treat infertility in PCOS. This medication is known as a selective estrogen receptor modulator and is typically prescribed for five days during the cycle, typically from Day 5 to Day 9. The standard starting dose is 50 mg per day. In many clinics, progesterone will be prescribed after ovulation to help promote implantation. The success rate of clomiphene is approximately ten percent per month for a woman with PCOS who is under thirty-seven years old. For women who ovulate regularly, the success rate is actually only one percent higher than trying naturally.

Clomiphene works by blocking estrogen receptors in the hypothalamus, which is the hormone control center of the brain. With these receptors blocked, the hypothalamus and pituitary gland are tricked into believing that estrogen is low, and they try to make more by stimulating the ovary to produce an egg. If a woman does not ovulate on 50 mg of clomiphene, it is often increased by 50 mg increments during subsequent cycles.

For a medication, clomiphene also has a very long half-life of approximately seven days. That means that only half of the medication will be excreted in a week, resulting in a good amount of it lingering in the system for some time, particularly if cycles are done back-to-back.

Side Effects

Common side effects can include temporary enlargement of the ovaries as well as hot flashes. Some women also experience mood changes, psychiatric concerns, GI effects, breast discomfort, and visual disturbances. Unfortunately, clomiphene also has some anti-fertility effects, including thinning the endometrial lining and drying up cervical mucus, which is not ideal.

Clomiphene is also associated with an increased risk of multiple births. Overall, the chances of conceiving twins on clomiphene is around seven percent, with a one percent chance of conceiving higher-order multiples, such as triplets or quadruplets. Multiple pregnancies are at higher risk than single pregnancies and can be particularly risky in women with PCOS who may have other complicating factors, such as gestational diabetes.

Conventional Medications for PCOS Fertility Treatment

- Clomiphene
- Letrozole
- Gonadotrophins
- Metformin
- Progesterone
- Low-dose aspirin
- Immune-modulating medication

Success of Clomiphene

Clomiphene does not appear to be very successful in women who ovulate normally, with only a five percent success rate per cycle (compared to four percent without). In women who have difficulty ovulating, the pregnancy success rate is much higher, ranging from ten to thirty percent. For women who do not have fertility problems, the chance of conceiving on any one cycle is around ten to twenty-five percent.

Many clinics recommend that a couple not complete more than three consecutive clomiphene cycles due to its long half-life as well as the fact that eighty-five percent of successful clomiphene cycles occur within the first three cycles. To make it short, if it doesn't work in three cycles, it's pretty unlikely to work after that, and the negative effects may outweigh success. Some clinics, however, will do up to six consecutive cycles.

Letrozole

Letrozole is a medication that is used off-label for fertility purposes. It is actually a medication that has been developed for the treatment of postmenopausal breast cancer, but doctors have found that it can also trigger ovulation if used in a similar way to clomiphene. Letrozole blocks what is known as aromatase, which is an enzyme that converts testosterone to estrogen. As such, the brain perceives a low level of estrogen and then hopefully stimulates ovulation.

Side Effects

Letrozole appears to have a lower side effect profile than clomiphene, as it is excreted much more quickly, and its overall action is different. A Canadian study that was presented at the American Association for Reproductive Medicine Conference in 2005 suggested that there was an increased risk of birth defects for women using letrozole.[1] This was countered later by a more detailed follow-up study that found it, in fact, caused a lower rate of congenital malformations (2.4 percent) and chromosomal abnormalities than clomiphene's 4.8 percent.[2]

Progesterone

Progesterone is often added to medicated cycles after ovulation, as it helps to prepare the lining for implantation. This is particularly important for women with PCOS, since many have low progesterone-to-estrogen ratios. This low ratio occurs because the first half of the cycle is typically longer than the second half, resulting in a relative excess of estrogen to progesterone.

Progesterone is particularly important in IVF because after the follicles are retrieved from the ovary, the corpus luteum isn't able to produce enough progesterone because it is punctured when the eggs are retrieved. As such, very high doses of progesterone, such as 400+ mg per day, may be commonly used in women with PCOS who are undergoing in vitro fertilization (IVF).

Immune-Modulating Medications

For patients who have had recurrent miscarriages or implantation failures, some doctors are now prescribing medications to calm the immune system. These include steroids, such as dexamethasone; anti-clotting agents (aspirin or low molecular weight heparin, for instance); and immune modulators (such as IVIG, intralipids, or lymphocyte immunization therapies). One common side effect of immune suppressants in particular is an increased risk of infection. For anti-clotting agents, there is an increased risk of bleeding.

Gonadotropins

Gonadotropins are injectable fertility drugs that can stimulate ovulation. These stronger drugs are often used when a woman does not respond to, or achieve pregnancy after, clomiphene or letrozole. Gonadotropins are actually forms of FSH and LH, which are the same hormones that are produced by the pituitary gland to stimulate the ovary naturally. Injections usually begin on Day 3 or 4 of the menstrual cycle and last approximately eight to ten days. During injections, patients are carefully monitored through bloodwork and ultrasound to determine the number of follicles and the staging of ovulation.

Once it appears that ovulation is imminent, patients are given a "trigger shot" of human chorionic gonadotropin (hCG) to stimulate ovulation. At this point, intra-uterine insemination (IUI) is often performed. These same medications are also used in IVF, which is a more involved process. In IVF, after the trigger shot causes the eggs to mature, they are extracted from the ovary and fertilized and then reimplanted into the uterus.

Side Effects

As injectable gonadotropins are much more direct and powerful than medications such as clomiphene, many more follicles will mature during the cycle. In women with PCOS, who often have an abundance of follicles in the first place, gonadotropins are even more risky.

Women with PCOS are at increased risk for ovarian hyperstimulation syndrome (OHSS) and may produce a large number of follicles on stimulation. OHSS can be a serious condition resulting in severe abdominal water retention and even hospitalization, so women with PCOS must be monitored carefully when using gonadotropins. In women with PCOS, a GnRH agonist called leuprolide is often used to stimulate ovulation instead of hCG, as it reduces risks of hyperstimulation syndrome. Coasting is another method used to prevent OHSS in women with PCOS undergoing IVF. In coasting, gonadotropins are stopped at a certain point, allowing follicles to "coast" and estradiol levels to calm before the trigger shot.

The risk of twins and even triplets or higher-order multiples is also greatly increased with gonadotropins, particularly when IUI is used. This is because in an IVF cycle, one embryo can be selectively transferred back into the uterus. In an IUI with injectables, all eggs that have matured will have the opportunity to be fertilized. As such, women with PCOS are often prescribed very low doses of gonadotropins during an IUI cycle.

Metformin

Metformin is also commonly used during fertility treatment for women with PCOS. It can be used as a stand-alone treatment, as research suggests that it may increase the number of natural ovulations in women with PCOS. Metformin works by increasing insulin sensitivity, hence reducing the harmful effects of high insulin on the ovary. That said, metformin may not translate into live births and take-home babies. In most trials on this subject, clomiphene and metformin were combined, and in the women taking metformin, there was only a slightly increased rate of live births. However, to counter, there was also an increased rate of miscarriage in metformin groups. As mentioned before, metformin may interfere with one-carbon metabolism and mitochondrial function, and therefore more research needs to be done to fully understand its effects on fetal development. As discussed in chapter 3, the most common side effects of metformin are gastrointestinal, including cramping, nausea, and loose stools.

Fertility Procedures

We have discussed the medications used in conventional fertility care. Now, I'll outline what happens during the most common fertility clinic procedures for women with PCOS.

IUI

Intrauterine insemination is when washed sperm are injected directly into a woman's uterus. To wash sperm, the sample is taken and individual sperm are separated from the seminal fluid. This helps to remove any dead or unhealthy sperm, mucus, or white blood cells. Also, in order to inject the sperm into the uterus, the seminal fluid must be removed, as it contains prostaglandins that can cause cramping. Normally, the cervix will filter out much of the prostaglandins.

IUI can be useful if there is any issue with male-factor infertility. It can be done naturally or teamed up with medications, such as clomiphene or gonadotropins. As mentioned previously, IUI may not be performed on a woman with PCOS if injectables are given, as there may be multiple follicles that have matured and the risk of multiples would be much higher.

IVF

You've probably heard quite a lot about IVF, as it's definitely the most popular and well-known fertility procedure. IVF involves the use of gonadotropins (injectables) to help the ovary produce multiple follicles and eggs (see Figure A-5). The follicles are then retrieved from the ovary through the wall of the vagina while the patient is under sedation.

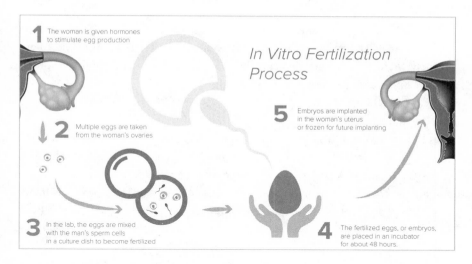

Figure A-5: The IVF Process

The eggs are then fertilized in the laboratory and matured for either three or five days. This is where the term "test-tube baby" came from. After the embryos have developed, they are then transferred selectively back to the uterus.

Most modern clinics will do a single embryo transfer to reduce the likelihood of twins and multiple births, but in cases where there has not been success in the past, or when the embryo quality does not look ideal, more than one embryo may be transferred.

During IVF, embryos are graded on their quality, which is decided upon by the number of cells and overall structure. An embryo that has developed to five days and has reached the stage known as blastocyst is considered to have the best chance of success in implantation.

Natural Fertility Treatments for PCOS

Now we enter the fascinating world of how to treat subfertility in PCOS naturally. Note that I said subfertility, rather than infertility. In almost all cases, women with PCOS can conceive. It simply takes the right treatment.

As is always the case, the first step is to address nutrition and lifestyle. As outlined in chapter 9, women with PCOS often do best eating foods that create lower insulin responses and on a plan that is high in vegetable intake and moderate in high-quality lean proteins and healthful fats. This way of eating lowers insulin levels, reducing any harmful impact on the ovaries. Exercise is also a helpful strategy for women with PCOS who are trying to conceive. I often recommend a moderate strength-training program three to four times per week.

In many cases, treatment with nutrition and exercise are all that is needed for women with PCOS to be able to conceive. In other cases, it may not be enough. Fortunately, there are some supplements that can be exceptionally helpful for women with PCOS when it comes to getting pregnant.

Inositol Complexes

Inositols are profoundly important for women with PCOS who are trying to conceive. Studies have suggested that inositol plays a crucial role in cell growth and development. Myo-inositol regulates the secretion from glands, such as the ovaries, and may be responsible for important signals essential for egg development. Numerous studies have confirmed that the presence of myo-inositol in the follicular fluid has a positive correlation with egg quality and maturation, particularly for women with PCOS.[3]

When it comes to fertility, inositol has been involved in some fascinating research in the PCOS world. A study published in 2012 in the *Archives of Gynecology and Obstetrics* found that a combination of D-chiro-inositol (DCI) and myo-inositol in a ratio of 1 to 40 was able to improve egg quality and pregnancy rates in women with PCOS undergoing IVF.[4]

Overall, it has been found that myo-inositol can improve ovarian responsiveness to the natural hormones FSH and LH that are made by a woman's pituitary gland and can help to reestablish timely ovulation. This can increase the chances of a spontaneous pregnancy. Other research has found that myo-inositol is simply an excellent "ovary vitamin," as it can improve follicle health and implantation rates during IVF cycles for women without PCOS as well.[5]

I can recall one patient in particular, Suzanne, a twenty-seven-year-old woman with PCOS, who after trying to conceive for over a year began on a course of myo-inositol and swiftly became pregnant within just two months. She was amazed at how quickly it worked for her and at how relaxed she felt with the treatment. Myo-inositol has another wonderful benefit: It reduces anxiety. This is always helpful for those on the stress-inducing infertility journey.

The inositols are generally very well tolerated. Rare side effects can include mild gastrointestinal upset and/or loose stool.

DCI

D-chiro-inositol (DCI) has been used in combination with myo-inositol for the treatment of infertility. It seems that DCI has quite a beneficial effect on insulin resistance in PCOS. A study looking at fifty-four women with PCOS provided increasing doses of DCI, ranging from 300 to 2,400 mg of DCI.

Unfortunately, however, women in the groups receiving the three highest DCI doses had poorer egg quality and lower-quality embryos in fertility treatment.[6] As such, and as the study noted above suggests, DCI may be best utilized in fertility patients at lower doses. That being said, it appears that DCI is, in fact, a beneficial product for women with PCOS who are trying to conceive, particularly when used in the recommended doses. DCI is generally very well tolerated. Rare side effects can include mild gastrointestinal upset and/or loose stool.

Combined Inositol Therapy

It's currently thought that the optimal ratio of myo-inositol to DCI for fertility may be 40:1. This is the ratio found in plasma. This specific ratio appears to be more effective than either myo-inositol or DCI alone when it comes to metabolic health and ovulatory function without negatively impacting oocyte health. This would be the equivalent of 4 grams of myo-inositol along with 100 mg of D-chiro-inositol per day, often in two divided doses.

N-Acetyl Cysteine

N-acetyl cysteine (NAC) is another supplement that has been researched for the treatment of PCOS-related infertility. NAC is a compound that comes from the sulphur-containing amino acid L-cysteine and has been traditionally used to thin out mucus during bronchitis or other chest conditions. It has also been used in conventional medicine to prevent liver damage from alcohol and acetaminophen. This same compound has been researched for fertility in PCOS.

One of the first studies on NAC for fertility in PCOS was a 2005 study on women who previously did not ovulate when given clomiphene. Giving NAC to these women in addition to the clomiphene increased the rates of ovulation and pregnancy significantly.[7] Another study repeated this finding in 2012, discovering that in a group of 180 women with PCOS, 1.2 grams per day of NAC plus clomiphene improved the number of follicles retrieved, the thickness of the endometrial lining, and ovulation and pregnancy rates when compared to clomiphene alone.[8]

The reason that NAC seems to be such a powerful therapeutic treatment for PCOS lies in several properties. It is a powerful antioxidant and increases the amount of the master antioxidant glutathione produced in the ovary, which is crucial for fertility. It also increases insulin sensitivity, is anti-inflammatory, and reduces serum testosterone levels and the free-androgen index.[9] Women with high androgens, anovulation, insulin resistance, and inflammation can all benefit from NAC.

Side Effects

Rare side effects of NAC are heartburn, nausea, or changes in bowel movements. Many patients find that taking it with food is very helpful in preventing these side effects.

Vitamin D

Vitamin D is a crucial compound for women with PCOS who wish to achieve pregnancy. Although commonly known as a vitamin, it is actually an important hormone involved in many processes of the reproductive cycle. Vitamin D receptors have been found in the ovary, endometrium, and placenta. A deficiency of this hormone can even contribute to the arrested development of follicles in the ovary of women with PCOS, stopping ovulation. Mice whose vitamin D receptors have been genetically removed demonstrate severe abnormalities in the folliculogenesis process (the growth of the eggs).

In a study on 368 women undergoing IVF, the patients that were deficient in vitamin D had lower pregnancy rates.[10]

Deficiencies of vitamin D have been linked to alterations of LH and sex hormone-binding globulin, testosterone levels, insulin resistance, and serum insulin levels in women with PCOS. Women with deficiencies of this key vitamin have even been found to have close to half the success rate in IVF cycles compared to women with optimal vitamin D levels. Vitamin D receptors also play an important role in estrogen production in the ovary, and it is known that vitamin D deficiency is also linked very clearly to insulin resistance in PCOS.

So now that it's clear that women with PCOS need to have excellent vitamin D status in order to achieve pregnancy, my general recommendation is that women with this condition should have their vitamin D levels checked regularly. A goal for women with PCOS should be 50–70 ng/ml (or 124–175 nmol/l).

Forms of Vitamin D

The best form of vitamin D is vitamin D3, also known as cholecalciferol, which is the natural form of D that your body makes from sunlight. The vitamin D3 that is readily available is usually manufactured from sheep's lanolin, which provides the same type of vitamin D that your body manufactures. For deficient patients, 4,000 IU may be taken daily to restore levels.

Vitamin D2, which is often manufactured from a yeast source, is generally not as well absorbed as D3. Studies indicate that D2 is much less potent and has a shorter duration of action than vitamin D3. Overall, D3 has been estimated to be around three times as effective.

Historically, however, if a patient is severely deficient, single large doses of vitamin D can be prescribed in 50,000 IU capsules by a physician. Women with all expressions of PCOS should pay close attention to their vitamin D levels.

Side effects of vitamin D are extremely rare. However, it is not recommended to have levels above the reference range until there is more long-term data.

Berberine

Berberine is a newer compound to the PCOS fertility scene. It's an active component of several different plants ranging from barberry to goldenseal and is especially prominent in a variety of herbs rooted in the traditional Chinese medicine profession, such as *Rhizoma coptidis* and phyllodendron. In traditional Chinese medicine, berberine has been used to improve insulin resistance and treat diabetes for centuries. Modern studies have suggested that berberine actually has an action similar to metformin as an insulin sensitizer. Now, research suggests that this compound may also have an application for PCOS-related infertility.

A 2013 study on 150 women with PCOS who were undergoing IVF investigated the use of berberine. In this trial, the groups of women were placed either on metformin, berberine, or a placebo. Both metformin and berberine similarly improved the pregnancy rate and reduced ovarian hyperstimulation syndrome. Berberine did even better: It specifically improved live birth rate as well.[11] Overall, it appears that berberine may be a viable alternative to metformin for the treatment of infertility in women with PCOS and is particularly useful for women who suffer from insulin resistance or who are overweight. Side effects of berberine include gastrointestinal upset and loose stool.

Maitake Mushroom

Grifola frondosa (also known as maitake mushroom) is a mushroom that has many different medicinal uses. Apart from its powerful effects on the immune system, maitake is a useful treatment for PCOS-related infertility. In 2010, a study conducted on eighty Japanese patients with anovulatory PCOS found that *Grifola frondosa* induced an ovulation rate of 76.9 percent at a dose of 250 mg of dried maitake mushroom powder per tab, at a dose of 3 tabs 3 times daily between meals.[12] For patients who had previously been resistant to clomiphene, adding maitake to their regimes resulted in an ovulation rate of seventy-five percent.

Maitake's positive action on ovulation is thought to be from its effects on insulin resistance, which have been well researched, as it is commonly used for the treatment of diabetes. As such, it's very helpful for women with insulin resistance. Maitake mushroom is also well suited to women with high androgens, as it has been found to exert anti-androgenic effects.

Natural Progesterone Cream

Many women with PCOS have low progesterone levels, which commonly occurs due to poor follicle health and delayed ovulation. Overall, there is a relative excess of estrogen, given that the follicular phase is often quite lengthy, and the amount of progesterone supplied in the shorter luteal phase may not be enough to sustain a

pregnancy. As such, many women with PCOS find it helpful to use natural progesterone products that are available over the counter. It is important not to use these
products prior to ovulation, however, so a woman should be able to identify her ovulation timing before utilizing them. The cream is generally applied to the capillary
rich surfaces, such as the face, neck, chest, breasts, inner arms, or palms.

Rotate the area of application daily to avoid saturating the same area with the
cream. It is very important to cycle progesterone on and off, unless specifically prescribed by your doctor, to avoid creating a continuously high level of progesterone,
which could inhibit ovulation. Natural progesterone cream can be used by women
who don't ovulate regularly or have luteal phase defects. It can also be used in women
who don't ovulate at all, but this is more complex and should be supervised by a
health-care practitioner. Finally, it can also be used in early pregnancy to assist in
preventing miscarriage. For women who have had or who have a family history of
female reproductive or breast cancers, all hormones should be used under strict
supervision of a physician.

Vitex Agnus-Castus

Vitex agnus-castus is a beautiful plant with some remarkable properties. Also known
as chaste tree or chasteberry, it is a very popular herb in women's health. As described
in detail in chapter 6, it is believed that vitex works primarily on the pituitary gland
and the opiate system in the brain.

Vitex is a plant that may be either beneficial or detrimental to women with PCOS
when it comes to fertility. There is some evidence that vitex can either reduce or increase
the amount of prolactin, depending on the dosage used. Typically, vitex is most effective when a woman has a higher-than-average prolactin level, as prolactin hinders
ovulation, disrupting the natural production of fertility-promoting progesterone.

Vitex is thought to be helpful for luteal phase defects, which are common in
PCOS. Luteal phase defects are the result of low progesterone levels. A weak luteal
phase from low progesterone can make it difficult for the embryo to implant successfully in the womb. In some cases, luteal phase defect may even be caused by
"hidden" elevated prolactin levels, also known as latent hyperprolactinemia. One
study found that in a group of fifty-two women with luteal phase defect due to latent
hyperprolactinemia, there was a significant increase in the length of the luteal phase
with vitex therapy.[13] As previously discussed, vitex can also act to slow the pulsing of
GnRH due to its effects on the hypothalamic neurons, a benefit for women who have
pituitary-related ovulatory problems.

With respect to dosing and more about indications, please see the detailed information on vitex in chapter 6.

Black Cohosh

Black cohosh (*Cimicifuga racemosa*) is an intriguing women's health botanical that provides clear benefits for the treatment of infertility in PCOS. An Egyptian study found that this cluster-flowered member of the buttercup family might be comparable to clomiphene in ovulation induction in women with PCOS. The study provided one group of women with black cohosh at 20 mg daily for ten days and a second group of women with clomiphene. The result for the cohosh group was similar to the clomiphene group with respect to FSH/LH ratios. Progesterone levels and endometrial thickness were both higher in the black cohosh groups. Most importantly, the pregnancy rate was also higher.[14]

Cohosh has also been combined with clomiphene in research, and it has been found to decrease some of the negative side effects associated with the drug, such as thin lining and scanty cervical mucus. In the groups where cohosh was combined with clomiphene, there was a thicker endometrial lining, increased progesterone, and an increased clinical pregnancy rate.[15]

Additionally, black cohosh possesses anti-inflammatory properties, which may be beneficial for PCOS. It's important to note that in some patients, however, black cohosh may raise liver enzymes. As such, if you are using this herb, you should be monitored by a physician or naturopath to ensure that you can tolerate it. If you have liver disease, black cohosh may not be a good choice for you. Black cohosh may be particularly helpful for patients who have female hormonal imbalance and ovulatory dysfunction as a stronger factor in their case.

Dosing of black cohosh for fertility is typically 20 mg per day from Day 1 to Day 10 of your cycle.

Resveratrol

Resveratrol is a natural polyphenol that is found in grapes, berries, nuts, and red wine. It has been widely studied for its benefits to the cardiovascular system and for its effects against cancer.

Resveratrol appears to stop the overgrowth of ovarian theca cells. In a PCOS ovary, there is an overgrowth of these testosterone-producing cells. These cells are involved in the enlarged, cystic appearance of the ovaries in PCOS, as they hinder ovulation. Resveratrol can regulate the overgrowth of theca cells, helping to normalize the structure and function of the ovary in women with PCOS.

It is also anti-inflammatory and reduces clotting, making it helpful for endometrial lining health and implantation. Typical dosages of trans-resveratrol range from 100 to 250 mg per day. Resveratrol can thin the blood, so it should not be combined with other blood thinners unless under the supervision of a doctor.

Coenzyme Q10

Coenzyme Q10 (CoQ10) is a mitochondrial antioxidant and is definitely one of the most popular supplements to treat infertility in general. The mitochondria are the powerhouses of the cell, and their health is crucial to the health of the oocytes. Healthy oocytes contain a good number of mitochondria with healthy DNA, and when an embryo is formed, the mitochondria from the mother are transferred to the embryo, whereas those from the sperm are not, meaning that mitochondrial health has a large role to play in the formation of a healthy embryo. Women with PCOS often have concerns about egg quality due to the impact of androgens and insulin resistance on their ovaries. Supporting the mitochondria may provide great benefits for the diminished ovarian health common in PCOS.

A study published in March of 2014 investigated the use of CoQ10 in 101 women who suffered with infertility from PCOS and were resistant to clomiphene treatment. The CoQ10 group had a greater number of mature follicles, better endometrial lining, and a much greater ovulation rate (65.9 percent compared to 15.5 percent in the control group). The pregnancy rate was also higher in the CoQ10 group (37.3 percent compared to six percent in the control group).[16]

Overall, this study concluded that CoQ10 was an effective treatment for women with PCOS who are resistant to clomiphene. CoQ10 may be beneficial for all phenotypes of PCOS who are trying to conceive, particularly for women over thirty-five years of age.

My personal preference when it comes to CoQ10 for fertility is to use the reduced form, ubiquinol. This is the anti-oxidant form of CoQ10 and may be better absorbed than its counterpart ubiquinone (as shown in Figure A-6).

Both nutrients, however, can provide benefits, as ubiquinone can be converted into ubiquinol. If you are only able to get CoQ10, rather than ubiquinol, you can use a higher dosage. I would typically recommend 600–800 mg per day of ubiquinone and 200–300mg per day of ubiquinol.

Side effects of CoQ10 are rare, but can include a mild reduction in blood pressure.

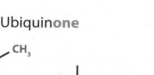
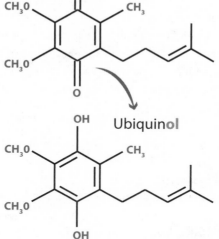

Figure A-6: Ubiquinone and Ubiquinol

Case Study

Moira was a forty-two-year-old lean woman with PCOS who ovulated regularly, yet suffered from hirsutism and anxiety. Despite being in her forties, she still had numerous small follicles on her ultrasounds. When Moira was younger, she had exceptionally high DHEA levels, but these had decreased with age. Moira had been trying to conceive for two years without any luck. After trying both IUI and IVF, she felt frustrated. Doctors told her that she appeared to have a good follicle count for her age, yet these eggs didn't seem to be of good quality. She was told that women with PCOS who are in their forties often retain more follicles but that the quality still declined with age.

After seeing Moira in the clinic, we found that her insulin levels were fairly normal; however, her vitamin D was exceptionally low. I began her on a regimen of 300 mg of ubiquinol for mitochondrial support, myo-inositol at 4 grams daily, and 5,000 IU of vitamin D per day. Knowing that focusing on her egg quality would be key, we also increased overall nutrition, including supplementing omega-3 fatty acids and following a whole-food, low insulin index, gluten-free diet. Within four months, Moira conceived naturally and carried to term a beautiful baby girl.

As we have learned, the follicles develop over many months prior to a cycle, which is why it takes several months to work on egg quality in women with PCOS. In Moira's case, she conceived once the cycles of folliculogenesis brought forth new, healthy follicles.

White Peony

White peony, or *Paeonia lactiflora*, is a mainstay in women's health in traditional Chinese medicine. White peony has been shown to lower androgen levels in vitro. A compound known as paeoniflorin inhibits the production of testosterone and promotes the aromatase enzyme that converts testosterone into estrogen.

Similarly to vitex, peony may be helpful in decreasing serum prolactin levels. Other research has found that peony, as part of a traditional Japanese medicine compound, helps to promote ovulation.[17]

Licorice Root

Often combined with peony for the treatment of PCOS, licorice has myriad fertility benefits. This herb is both anti-inflammatory and anti-androgenic.

A small trial found that licorice root significantly decreases testosterone levels in women. Licorice contains phytoestrogens, glycyrrhizin, and glycyrrhetic acid, which have a weak anti-androgenic effect. It also provides benefit for the adrenals. This herb is considered safe while trying to conceive, so it can be an excellent choice for women with PCOS who are experiencing infertility. It's important to note, however, that it should be used with caution, as it may increase blood pressure. Licorice is most beneficial for women with androgen excess. Peony and licorice formula is typically taken at a dosage of 2 grams 3 times per day, and up to 4 grams 3 times per day.

Maria, our woman with PCOS from the beginning of the chapter, came to see me after her three-year fertility journey. As she still wasn't ovulating regularly, we made some significant changes to her diet and exercise program and added some supplements and herbs. For Maria, we used peony root and licorice daily to

Anti-Androgenic	Paeonia Licorice Myo-inositol Grifolia Resveratrol NAC Omega 3 Fatty Acid Vitamin D
Ovulation Promoting	Myo-inositol DCI NAC Paeonia Licorice Progesterone CoQ10 Grifolia Black Cohosh Vitamin D Vitex Resveratrol
Insulin Resistance	DCI Myo-inositol NAC Resveratrol Berberine Vitamin D
Stress/Adrenal	Licorice Paeonia Vitex Myo-inositol
Inflammation	Resveratrol Grape seed Extract Licorice
Thyroid	Iodine (low dose only) Selenium Tyrosine

Table A-1: Natural Fertility Treatments by Factor

regulate her hormones and improve ovulation. She also took berberine to reduce insulin resistance and myo-inositol for its many benefits. Following the diet for insulin resistance outlined in chapter 9, Maria was able to lose ten inches from her waist and twenty pounds. Over time, her cycles began to shorten and regulate. After only six months, she became pregnant. Nine months later, she delivered an adorable baby boy named William.

Acupuncture

There is a good deal of research on the use of acupuncture to treat infertility in PCOS, much of which has been conducted by Elisabet Stener-Victorin from Sweden, an avid researcher on the effects of acupuncture on PCOS. Studies have found that among other benefits, electroacupuncture may decrease the overabundant nerve growth factor that occurs in PCOS, increase the rate of ovulation, and improve androgens in women with PCOS, which have clear benefits for fertility.[18, 19]

Inflammation

As we already know, women with PCOS have increased inflammation either in their bloodstream, within the ovary itself, or in other organs of the body, such as the liver. Inflammation is definitely detrimental for fertility. In the earliest stages of pregnancy, it's important to enter into a calmer type of immunological state. Many women catch colds and flus in the early stages of pregnancy, and this is because the immune system down-regulates its function at that time, allowing the embryo to implant successfully.

With PCOS, women may have more challenges entering into this state, and as such, the immune system may not be in the most optimal situation for conception. Studies have found that women with PCOS have higher circulating levels of inflammatory mediators like C-reactive protein, TNF-alpha, and PAI-1. Treatment of insulin resistance can reduce these inflammatory mediators, and it's also possible to affect them directly with anti-inflammatory treatments. Miscarriage rates are increased in PCOS, possibly as a result of localized inflammation and insulin resistance or poor egg quality, which is a result of the disorder.

Grape seed extract and pine bark offer a decrease in the TH1-dominant inflammatory responses that can cause difficulty with implantation of an embryo. A high quality omega-3 fatty acid, in addition to its benefits for reducing testosterone, can also mitigate inflammation.

Fish oils are often best sourced from small fish, such as anchovies and sardines. Research also suggests that fish oil can lower androgen levels and should be used in women who have high levels of these hormones. Triglyceride forms of fish oils that are molecularly distilled to remove all heavy metals and environmental toxins are likely the best choice. Also look for a fish oil company that posts their third party batch testing results. For more information on anti-inflammatory approaches, please see chapter 2.

MTHFR

Women with PCOS who are trying to conceive should be checked for mutations in the methylenetetrahydrofolate reductase (MTHFR) gene, as it can be an additional complicating factor in fertility if present. Women with PCOS are particularly susceptible to MTHFR mutations, as the underlying metabolic condition can be additive with its effects.

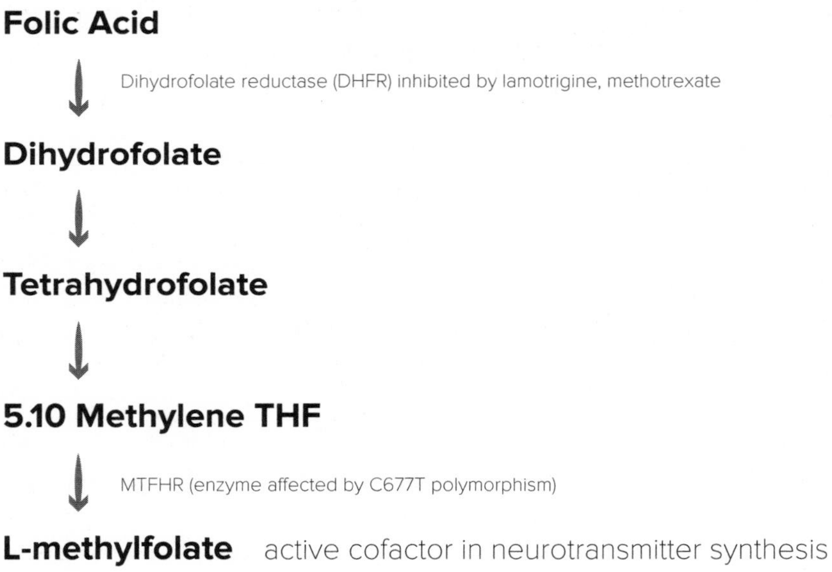

Folic Acid

↓   Dihydrofolate reductase (DHFR) inhibited by lamotrigine, methotrexate

Dihydrofolate

↓

Tetrahydrofolate

↓

5.10 Methylene THF

↓   MTFHR (enzyme affected by C677T polymorphism)

L-methylfolate   active cofactor in neurotransmitter synthesis

Figure A-7: Conversion of Folic Acid to Methylfolate Impaired by Mutations in MTHFR

MTHFR can be associated with clotting and recurrent miscarriages, something common in PCOS. A mutation in MTHFR makes it difficult to convert folic acid into methylfolate, the form directly used in DNA repair and cell growth. Up to forty percent of people have a mutation in MTHFR. There are two different variants, MTHFR C677T and MTHFR A1298C. Of the two, the C677T causes a more serious problem in converting folic acid into methylfolate and is more highly associated with pregnancy losses.

If you are unable to get testing for MTHFR (see Resources section in Appendix E), it's important to ensure that you are taking a prenatal vitamin that contains the type of folate that is active and can be used by cells even if you do have this mutation. L-5-methylfolate is the preferred source of folate for women with PCOS who are trying to conceive. In addition, as mentioned in chapter 3, metformin affects one-carbon metabolism and methylation, so extra precaution should be taken for women who have MTHFR and are taking metformin.

Case Study

Sheri had Type 2 PCOS and a strong family history of high blood pressure and strokes. She had recurrent miscarriages, having experienced four, all of them quite early in pregnancy. On a subsequent pregnancy, after learning that she was homozygous for MTHFR C677T (the most severe form of MTHFR), she was able to carry the baby to term with the help of L-5 methyltetrahydrofolate and some gentle anti-clotting therapy: in her case, omega-3 fish oil.

Fertility-Safe Supplements for Women with PCOS and Thyroid Concerns

For a thorough description of supplements for women who have problems with thyroid health, please see chapter 7. Subclinical hypothyroidism or sluggish thyroid function can increase the risk for miscarriage and developmental problems with babies.

As is generally recommended for women with PCOS, the American Thyroid Association recommends that TSH should be below 2.5 miU/ml for the first trimester. Some of the therapeutics mentioned in chapter 7 are not suitable for women who are trying to conceive. Table A-1 offers a listing of fertility-safe thyroid treatments; however, please consult with a practitioner on their suitability for your case.

Infertility and Self Esteem

Infertility is a very stressful condition. It involves facing the potential loss of motherhood and all of the dreams that go along with life as a mother. Infertility also erodes our self-esteem and even our inherent value as women. Most girls grow up dreaming of being a mother, and when a woman learns that she may not be able to bring children into this world, it can be devastating. I would tell you to reach out and get all of the support that you can as you go through this difficult journey, whether that be through joining support groups or through a trusted counselor or therapist.

Although having children is a very real and important dream, fertility can have meaning beyond that of bringing a child into existence. My teacher Dr. Randine Lewis says, "You can give birth to any number of wonderful things in this world with your creative gifts." For women struggling with their fertility, reconnecting with the feminine, creative forces within can give back part of what we feel has been lost.

Many women find that embarking on a creative project such art, writing, crafting, or a new creative business venture can provide a great deal of emotional healing as they navigate this challenging terrain.

You Are Not Infertile

Overall, the picture can be quite complex for a woman with PCOS who is attempting to get pregnant, depending on her individual characteristics. It's important to keep in mind that the vast majority of women with PCOS do have the ability to conceive, although the process often takes awhile longer.

Like Maria, Sheri, or Moira, the right treatment is often the boost that is needed to help a woman with PCOS get and stay pregnant. I always tell my patients that PCOS is associated with subfertility, rather than infertility. Stay hopeful, no matter how long you've been trying. Most women with PCOS can and do achieve pregnancy!

PCOS and Pregnancy

Mary had suffered many years while trying to conceive due to difficulties associated with her PCOS. She went through years of fertility treatment and finally achieved her goal after three miscarriages. She wanted this pregnancy to be as healthy as possible. Mary had always struggled with her weight and had managed to lose twenty pounds before becoming pregnant. She was worried that pregnancy would cause her to gain all of this weight back. She also worried about gestational diabetes, knowing that diabetes ran in her family history. She didn't have any friends who had PCOS who were pregnant, so she came into the clinic to see what she could do to stay healthy. With the right diet, exercise, and nutritional program, she was able to have a healthy pregnancy carried to term and gave birth to a beautiful little baby girl.

Insulin Resistance in Pregnancy

Women with PCOS are commonly insulin resistant. This insulin resistance continues on in pregnancy, creating a variety of problems. We will go through the most common PCOS-related complications of pregnancy and the postpartum period and, most importantly, what you can do about them.

Supplements to support pregnancy in PCOS include—

- A quality prenatal vitamin, including methylfolate and around 30 mg of iron, along with a full spectrum of micronutrients, such as zinc, selenium, magnesium and B vitamins
- 3,000 IU of vitamin D, taken daily
- Omega-3 fatty acids, taken daily, including 500mg of DHA

- Calcium and magnesium (These should be taken separately from your prenatal vitamin. Bedtime is an excellent time for these supplements. I often recommend adding 800 mg of calcium and 400 mg of magnesium daily or more to achieve a total of 1,200 mg calcium and 600mg magnesium per day, including your dietary intake of these nutrients.)

Miscarriages

Even after all of the challenges you've gone through to conceive, the threat of miscarriage can continue to loom for women with PCOS. It's thought that the rate of miscarriage in PCOS can be close to double that of a typical pregnancy. The causes of miscarriage are thought to be linked to elevated insulin levels, which increase the risk of blood clotting—this can make delivering blood flow through the placenta a challenge. Some researchers have also found that the elevated androgens found in women with PCOS may be a culprit in miscarriage. It's thought that the hormonal and metabolic dysregulations found in PCOS can alter the uterine lining and the way that the embryo implants. Another highly prevalent factor is egg quality—in the presence of inflammation and oxidative stress, egg health can be compromised, increasing the risk of miscarriage.

What can you do to prevent miscarriage if you have PCOS?
The first thing you should do is follow all 8 steps prior to becoming pregnant, in order to produce healthier eggs and a healthier reproductive and metabolic environment. Importantly, you can also continue the PCOS diet program in pregnancy, with a slightly higher amount of carbohydrates with each meal. Typically, you can increase your starchy vegetable intake to the size of one handful with each meal, and then have "mini meal" snacks, three times daily.

Systemic Enzymes
One German trial on 144 women with immunologically mediated recurrent miscarriages treated with systemic enzymes in pregnancy produced promising results, as 114 of the women were able to carry healthy babies to term with this therapy. More research should be completed on this treatment, and it should not be used without the supervision of a physician. Systemic enzymes also have blood-thinning action and should not be combined with other anticoagulant medications unless prescribed by a physician.

EPA and Omega-3 Fatty Acids
In chapter 2, I spoke about using an EPA-dominant, molecularly distilled omega-3 fatty acid. This is an excellent way to reduce inflammation and insulin resistance in

pregnancy. I aim for a dosage of approximately 1,200 mg EPA and 500 mg DHA for pregnant women.

Low-Dose Aspirin

In many reproductive medicine clinics, low-dose (baby) aspirin is commonly recommended to thin the blood and prevent miscarriage. This should be done only with a doctor's supervision and should not be combined with any other blood-thinning agents without the close supervision of a health-care professional. Typically, the risk of miscarriage is minimal after twelve weeks. After this point, you may do best shifting back to the general pregnancy recommendations.

Gestational Diabetes

This is a common condition that women with PCOS are at increased risk for. Given that we have genetic predispositions to diabetes, it makes sense that gestational diabetes would be a risk we face as well. In particular, women over thirty-five have increased insulin resistance in pregnancy. Combine that with PCOS, and there is often gestational diabetes in older women as a result. The main risk of gestational diabetes is that it can cause your baby to grow too large. If the baby is too large, he or she will be at increased risk for a difficult birth or cesarean section.

It's best to check for gestational diabetes around twenty-seven weeks of gestation. This is routinely done with an oral glucose tolerance test. If your readings come back showing you are at risk for gestational diabetes, you can also check your own fasting and post-meal glucose at home with a glucometer. Check your blood sugar two hours after eating and aim for levels below 6.7 mmol/l (approximately 120 mg/dl). When it comes to fasting glucose in the morning, you should aim for below 5.8 mmol/l (105 mg/dl). If a meal causes your blood sugar to spike, look closely at the contents. Did you consume a carbohydrate-heavy meal? Was there hidden sugar in the meal? Did you have enough protein and vegetables with the meal to slow down the absorption of food?

Following your PCOS nutrition plan is the best way to combat gestational diabetes. Insulin counting isn't usually necessary: Simply structure your plate well, avoid sugar and excessive carbohydrates, and increase your vegetable intake. In addition, exercise can be a powerful weapon against this problem. There are many pregnancy-safe exercise videos available currently, and brisk walking or swimming is always an excellent form of exercise in pregnancy.

Fortunately, gestational diabetes almost always goes away immediately after delivering. However, having it does increase your future risk for diabetes, something women with PCOS are already quite aware of, unfortunately.

Some other tips that can help manage gestational diabetes include the following:

1. Increase fiber with your meals. Eat more vegetables with your meals or consider taking 10 grams of a fiber supplement from glucomannan/konjac root with a glass of water prior to each meal.

2. Myo-inositol has been studied for the prevention of gestational diabetes for women with PCOS. Taking 2 grams per day reduced the rate of gestational diabetes and high blood pressure by around half in a group of obese pregnant women.[20] This should be taken only under the supervision of a physician in pregnancy.

3. Never eat carbohydrates alone: Always combine them with a healthy fat or protein to slow their absorption.

Hypertension in Pregnancy

Women with PCOS are also at risk for hypertension in pregnancy. This is related to both insulin resistance and to the inflammatory environment created by the condition. This condition is also known as preeclampsia and can progress to a serious health condition for both mother and child. The chronic high blood pressure can restrict the blood flow to the baby through the placenta and can result in dangerous blood-clotting cascades in the mom. Like gestational diabetes, this condition resolves once you have had your baby. However, it puts you at risk for hypertension later on in life. Routine monitoring of protein in the urine as well as blood pressure is one of the ways that preeclampsia is picked up.

What can you do about hypertension during pregnancy? The following tips will help:

1. Continue to follow a healthy diet and exercise regularly.

2. Vitamin D levels should be checked and kept in the optimal range. Vitamin D deficiency has been linked to hypertension.

3. Magnesium is an excellent supplement that can be safely used in pregnancy. Magnesium citrate, at doses of 400–600 mg per day, is often helpful in both preventing and treating hypertension. In hospitals, IV magnesium is often used in hypertensive episodes and preeclampsia to reduce blood pressure.

4. Coenzyme Q10 has been studied for the prevention of preeclampsia at a dosage of 200 mg per day from twenty weeks of pregnancy to delivery. It was found that women on coenzyme Q10 had nearly half the rate of preeclampsia of women in the control group. This should be taken only under the supervision of a physician.

5. In some cases, pharmaceutical interventions may be required, so work closely with your doctor to keep your condition under control.

Postpartum Issues for Women with PCOS

Once baby has arrived, women with PCOS may face a few different issues in the postpartum period. This section will outline these and provide solutions to help you adjust to your new life with baby!

Breastfeeding

You've had your baby and everything went well. Congratulations! Many women with PCOS can breastfeed their newborn wonderfully and without any issues whatsoever, but there are some women who do have some challenges with breastfeeding due to PCOS. That being said, try not to worry until you see how it goes for you, since the majority of women with PCOS can breastfeed successfully!

There are a few reasons that some women with PCOS have trouble with breast-feeding. As teenage girls, there can be high levels of androgens and insufficient female hormones, such as estrogen, to develop the breast glandular tissue. Women with PCOS may have less glandular and more fatty tissues in their breasts or have small "tubular" breasts that are not well developed. In other cases, however, breast development isn't affected at all, and there are many women with PCOS who make ample milk and have a very easy time with breastfeeding.

The most important thing is to be gentle with yourself as you enter into your role as a new mom. Encouragement and support are important, so avoid anyone who makes you feel shame or guilt when you have tried your best.

To learn more, there are websites in the Resources section with tips on proper latching, compressions, and other important information you'll need in order to have your most optimal breastfeeding relationship with your child.

Good nutrition and keeping insulin resistance at bay are important for the support of breastfeeding in women with PCOS. You'll need more calcium and magnesium, and a supplement that has 1,000 mg of calcium and 500 mg of magnesium is often helpful.

You can continue to follow your PCOS nutrition recommendations, but you'll need an extra three hundred to five hundred calories per day, so try to achieve your additional needs with some extra lean protein and healthy fats, rather than loading up too much on the carbohydrates.

Batch cooking on the weekend is a great practice while you are breastfeeding. You can prep meals for the slow cooker for the week that won't take up too much time while you are caring for baby. Find easy solutions that allow you to continue your healthy eating patterns. For example, buy pre-chopped veggies or salads that make it easy to include the foods that will best support your health and that of your baby.

You should also drink plenty of water and take good care of yourself. Caring for a young infant is stressful, and the lack of sleep can disrupt your cortisol patterns, which can impact breastfeeding. Allow yourself breaks when possible, and find someone to cover for you while you nap.

Treatments to Improve Milk Supply

In some cases, herbal medicines can improve a milk supply that is struggling. You can try these, particularly if you are sure that you've addressed all issues with latch and supply-demand with a lactation consultant.

Herbal

Two herbs may be useful for women with PCOS who want to increase their milk supply. These are fenugreek and blessed thistle. Dr. Jack Newman of the International Breastfeeding Centre recommends taking three capsules of each, three times per day, and suggests that this should work within a day of starting them. Fenugreek should cause your skin to smell like maple syrup when taken in sufficient amounts.

Traditional

Domperidone is a medication that is prescribed to increase milk supply in women. It works by increasing the hormone prolactin, which stimulates milk production. It works by blocking dopamine receptors in the pituitary gland. There are some women for whom this is drug is contraindicated. This includes women who have any history of cardiac arrhythmia or anyone with chronic illness, abnormal liver function, or gastric abnormalities. As women with PCOS can be in these categories, they should always consult with an experienced physician to see if this medication may be safe for them.

Postpartum Depression and Anxiety

As women with PCOS have higher indices of depression and anxiety, the postpartum period may be a trigger for the onset of these conditions. Hormones, including progesterone, estrogen, and prolactin, are very high during pregnancy. Postpartum there is a huge crash of hormones, which can trigger mood disorders in many women. Be on the lookout for changes in your mood, lack of motivation, anxiety, or feeling unhappy with your role as a new mother.

If you aren't feeling quite right after having your baby, the most important thing is to reach out for support. Accept help from your family and friends, and get counseling if your feelings are out of control. Some supplements that are generally safe to take when breastfeeding include—

- B complex vitamin
- Magnesium
- Myo-inositol*

*This supplement can help with anxiety and is also beneficial for PCOS.

Postpartum Thyroid Dysfunction

The first four to six months after having a baby is the most likely time for problems to begin with thyroid function. As Hashimoto's thyroiditis (autoimmune thyroiditis) is more common in women with PCOS, it's important to look out for postpartum thyroiditis, an inflammatory condition that attacks the thyroid gland after having a baby. Therefore, be sure to check your thyroid antibodies six weeks after having a baby, particularly if you are feeling cold, tired, depressed, and are not able to lose weight.

Return of the Menses

Women with PCOS may have a longer period of what is known as postpartum amenorrhea, meaning that the time for the period to return is longer than for other women. This is related to the androgen excess and insulin resistance of the disorder. The best way to help move this along is to go through the 8 steps to reverse your PCOS that are shared in this book.

Pregnancy and new motherhood is a wonderful time in your life. Although PCOS may present many challenges to this period, the vast majority of women recover well and have healthy pregnancies and postpartum periods with the right diet and treatments. So, most of all, enjoy your special time with baby!

Appendix B

PCOS AND MENOPAUSE

Know that you are the perfect age. Each year is special and precious,
for you shall only live it once. Be comfortable with growing older.
—LOUISE HAY

Although we often think of PCOS as a condition that women of reproductive age experience, it is in fact a complex endocrine disorder that goes well past the menopausal years. As the number of eggs in our ovaries reduces as we approach menopause, the amount of androgens from the ovary will naturally decline. This often results in an apparent improvement of the PCOS hormonal condition, with more regular ovulations.

Menopause is defined as the time in a woman's life when ovulation and the menstrual cycles end, typically occurring around the age of fifty. It's defined as one year since the last menstrual cycle.

Perimenopause

Prior to menopause, there are several years when hormones begin to change, as the ovaries' function begins to slow down. We have learned that the female hormones are produced primarily through the process of ovulation, and as the ability to produce follicles and hormones declines, the overall hormonal status of a woman will change dramatically.

The typical length of perimenopause is four years. It often begins as a shortening of cycles, with ovulations occurring closer together. The later part of perimenopause is characterized by skipped cycles and longer periods of amenorrhea, lasting more than three months. Early menopause can be induced by smoking or autoimmunity, or it can be genetic.

The Hormones in Menopause

During the menopausal transition, the egg quality and quantity is altered, resulting in major differences in the ability of the follicles to respond to signals from the pituitary. When stimulated, the ovary makes estrogen as a follicle begins to grow; however, the surges of luteinizing hormone (LH) can be insufficient to trigger the ovulatory process in the perimenopausal period of life. As a result, there are often "ups-and-downs" of estrogen, which can create intense symptoms. Over time, as the follicles become fewer in number and ovulations farther apart, estrogen levels decrease and progesterone levels become nonexistent.

The Onset of Menopause

The first factor that mediates the onset of menopause is the ovarian reserve—the number of follicles housing eggs within the ovary. As women with PCOS do tend to have a higher than average ovarian reserve, it's not surprising that they tend to go into menopause an estimated two years later than other women.[1]

During perimenopause, the follicle-stimulating hormone (FSH) levels begin to rise, as the pituitary gland has to make an extra strong effort to pull the follicles out of the ovary. Overall, with aging, the ovary produces less of a substance known as inhibin B. Without inhibin B, much more FSH must be used to grow a follicle in preparation for ovulation. As we know, in PCOS, FSH tends to be relatively low compared to LH, so this initial increase in FSH is part of why the cycles of women with PCOS tend to be more regular as they become older. Although LH levels rise simultaneously, the FSH rises much more in comparison, helping to mitigate the abnormal ratio of these two hormones typically seen in PCOS.

During perimenopause, estrogen levels, at least at first, remain the same or may even increase due to the extra push from FSH. As perimenopause progresses, however, and the follicles begin to struggle, they are no longer able to produce estrogen consistently, and levels fluctuate and eventually drop. This stage is basically a roller-coaster ride of estrogen ups and downs. In some cycles, progesterone may be normal, but on other cycles, it may be rather low. This leads to a condition of estrogen dominance in which estrogen is not sufficiently opposed with progesterone.

Menopause

After the final menstrual period, there are no more ovulations, and as a result, the ovary doesn't make progesterone. However, it does tend to make a smaller amount of other persistent hormones, such as androstenedione.

As menopause continues, there is a decrease in insulin sensitivity in all women, which clearly magnifies any insulin resistance in women with PCOS. In fact, it seems that women with PCOS are more prone to increased insulin resistance than other women after menopause. This is not surprising, given the other ways we see this threaded through our lives.

Menopause and Androgens

When a woman goes through menopause, the vast majority of her hormones come from her adrenal glands. With respect to androgen levels, and considering that the ovary produces one-fourth of the body's testosterone and sixty percent of the body's androstenedione, it's fairly clear that these are going to decline significantly. The adrenal, however, makes forty percent of the androstenedione and all of the DHEA-S hormones. And although the adrenal hormones decline with age, this is quite gradual. Thus, these androgenic hormones remain and predominate after menopause. Interestingly, after menopause, around fifty percent of women still produce smaller amounts of androgens from their ovaries!

So, although our androgens decline significantly and cycles become regular as we get older, women with PCOS continue to have higher levels of androgens through adulthood when compared to other women.

There is a shift, however, in the way that androgen excess is expressed past the menopausal transition (over fifty years of age). There's an increase in the free androgen index and free testosterone levels in women with PCOS. If you'll remember, we learned the testosterone-binding protein called sex hormone-binding globulin decreases when there is insulin resistance. Post-menopause, insulin resistance allows androgens to roam freely in the bloodstream, still able to impact our bodies in both positive and negative ways. Leptin levels are also affected by menopause, with increased amounts found in women once their menses have come to an end, again driven by the weight gain that typically happens in this time. As we know that women with PCOS have lower adiponectin, the protective substance secreted by our fat cells, we are predisposed to greater insulin resistance, leptin resistance, and weight gain after menopause. In addition, within one year of the final menstrual period, women experience an increase in total cholesterol and LDL. The hormonal shift is thought to drive this increase.

When it comes to postmenopausal androgens, research from the National Institute of Health found a significant association between postmenopausal androgen levels and cardiovascular events.[2] Along with the direct effects of insulin resistance, this may explain why women with PCOS past menopause are more prone to cardiovascular disease.

The Female Hormones of Menopause

Androgens are typically transformed into estrogen in the tissues of the body. This process changes profoundly as a woman becomes older. Overall, there is less estradiol and androstenedione in the bloodstream, but testosterone and estrone don't decrease in the same manner and instead become more predominant. As such, estrone is the main estrogen in menopausal women.

There is a temporary rise in DHEA-S levels during the late time of menopause, when women's periods start to become farther apart. As a result, women who have adrenal androgen excess can experience an even more marked irregularity with their periods and longer spans of menopausal transition before their periods ultimately stop.

Osteoporosis in Women with PCOS

Osteoporosis is a major concern for all women as they enter into the perimenopausal transition. But here's some good news: Numerous studies have found that women with PCOS may be protected from osteoporosis, due to increased androgen levels.[3] Androgens can stimulate bone growth in women with PCOS, increasing bone density throughout life. Women with PCOS also tend to have more lean muscle mass, which can also improve bone density.

However, on the flip side, women who have gone very long periods of time with low estrogen levels may be more at risk for osteoporosis. This is less common, however, since most women with PCOS still produce estrogen, even if they are not ovulating regularly. That being said, if you are in this category, it's very important to have yourself closely monitored.

Another concern with osteoporosis is that insulin resistance is associated with decreased vitamin D levels, which can reduce bone mineral density. So women should be especially vigilant about vitamin D postmenopause.

Options Available to Perimenopausal Women with PCOS

When entering the menopausal transition, most women can benefit from changing their nutritional and supplemental program. For those who have significant PCOS symptoms, there are some natural options that can ease discomfort during this time.

Hormonal Regulation

Some of the bothersome symptoms of perimenopause and menopause include hot flashes, night sweats, mood swings, vaginal dryness, loss of libido, insomnia, bloating, breast pain, and heavy menses. Some of these symptoms are the result of low levels of estrogen and progesterone, while others are the result of fluctuating roller-coaster-type hormones. For the hormonal symptoms of menopausal transition, women with PCOS have a few basic options.

Siberian Rhubarb

An extract from this plant known as ERr 731 has been found to significantly reduce symptoms in both peri- and postmenopausal women. This includes a reduction of the number of daily hot flashes on par with low dose hormone replacement therapy, and it may address a variety of other menopausal symptoms.

This herb does act on the estrogen receptor, and so it should not be used by any woman with any history of breast cancer. The typical dosage is 4 mg of ERr 731 per day.

Valerian Root

An herb that has been traditionally prescribed for insomnia, valerian has been found to be beneficial in menopause as well. One study followed seventy-six menopausal women with hot flashes. The treatment group took 225 mg of valerian three times per day. There was a significant improvement in severity and frequency of hot flashes after four weeks of treatment.[4]

Black Cohosh

Black cohosh, or *Cimicifuga racemosa*, is likely the most researched herbal medicine for menopause, having been studied extensively for the treatment of menopausal complaints like hot flashes and vaginal dryness. Long believed to have phytoestrogenic (plant-estrogen) activity, it is now thought that cohosh likely works through a different mechanism, as it does not appear to bind to estrogen receptors.[5]

Current findings on the mechanisms of black cohosh in the treatment of menopausal concerns point to its impacts on the brain—namely, to its effects on the hypothalamus through neurotransmitters. This correlates with what is currently thought to be involved in causing hot flashes. Estrogen influences the firing rate of neurons in areas of the brain that regulate temperature and can change venous blood flow and artery tone. It's been found that substances in black cohosh can bind to the same neurotransmitter receptors known to be involved in creating hot flashes.

As discussed previously, another benefit of black cohosh is that it has some anti-androgenic properties. It can inhibit 5 alpha-reductase, the enzyme that converts testosterone into the strong androgen DHT. As many women with PCOS continue to experience androgenic symptoms post menopause, this might be an additional benefit.

In some rare cases, black cohosh can elevate liver enzymes, so its use should be monitored by a physician. Until more research is completed on its mechanisms, it is also not recommended for women with any history of breast cancer. Typical doses of black cohosh for menopausal concerns are 40 mg of dried rhizome powder per day.

Osteoporosis Prevention

Peri- and postmenopausal women with PCOS should be on a good mineral formula, including an absorbable form of calcium, magnesium, vitamin D, and trace minerals. Although androgens may be protective, women with PCOS still experience declining estrogen levels and are more susceptible to vitamin D deficiency post-menopause. As such, bone health should be a priority.

If you are consuming a diet rich in leafy green vegetables and whole foods, a good osteoporosis prevention formula for women with PCOS should include calcium citrate or hydroxyapatite at a dose of 600–900 mg per day, depending on diet and needs.

These forms of calcium are well absorbed and tolerated. Studies have found that calcium hydroxyapatite is significantly more effective than forms like calcium carbonate when it comes to supporting bone mineral density.

Vitamin K2 1 (MK7 menaquinone)

MK7 is a bioactive form of vitamin K, which plays an important and long-underestimated role in bone metabolism, calcium utilization, and activity of osteo calcium, which binds calcium within the bone. MK7 has been found to increase bone strength and reduce age-related decline in bone mineral density in the thoracic vertebrae, femoral neck, and lumbar spine.[6]

Typical doses range from 45 mcg to 180 mcg per day. As vitamin K can have effects on blood clotting pathways and oral anticoagulants, it is important to consult your physician about supplementation if you are taking these drugs.

Vitamin D

This should be increased to meet sufficiency, as previously discussed. However, a standard bone-building approach should include 3,000 IU per day, and in many cases more, since vitamin D deficiency is so common.

Silicon

Dietary silicon has been associated with good bone mineral density, as silicon is involved in collagen synthesis, bone mineralization, and connective tissue integrity. One trial found that added silicon in the form of choline-stabilized orthosilicic acid improved bone formation markers and femoral neck scores when added to a standard regiment of calcium and vitamin D.[7] Typical doses of silicon are in the range of 3 mg per day.

Exercise is always key for women with PCOS and during menopausal transition is no different. In fact, exercise becomes even more important at this time, when insulin resistance becomes more predominant.

It goes without saying that continuing to work on metabolic health through nutrition should come to the forefront as you make your transition into menopause. Please read through Appendix C to learn more about long-term cardiovascular and metabolic approaches, as well as chapters 2 and 3, which include detailed approaches on how to address insulin resistance and inflammation.

OBESITY, DIABETES, CANCER, AND CARDIOVASCULAR DISEASE IN PCOS

*The prevention of disease today is one of the most import-
ant factors in the line of human endeavor.*
—CHARLES MAYO

Amina was thirty-one years old and had suffered from PCOS since she was a teen-ager. She was an attractive woman with a silky brown bob and a successful job in a large financial company. She had been dating the same boyfriend for the past five years, and they hoped to start their family soon. Due to the pressures of her job and working long hours at the office, she had never been able to find much time to exercise and ate takeout food quite often. Many of her family members carried extra weight around their abdomens and had diabetes and high blood pressure. Amina went in for her annual physical exam and was shocked at what her doctor presented to her.

She was told that she had high triglycerides, high "bad" cholesterol, and high liver enzymes. The doctor then ordered an ultrasound and found that fatty tissue was beginning to engulf her liver. Amina thought she was too young for this. However, with PCOS these problems can start early, so it's important to monitor your health regularly.

Metabolic Risk Factors: Insulin Resistance and Type 2 Diabetes

PCOS makes it far more common to have metabolic risk factors, such as insulin resistance, high cholesterol, high blood pressure, and type 2 diabetes, putting us at much more risk for chronic disease.

As we've learned, the genes for PCOS are energy-conserving genes, and they've done us well in times of famine and physical stress. That being said, the standard Western diet does not work well with our genetics and provides the perfect environment for chronic disease to develop.

How Insulin Resistance Turns into Type 2 Diabetes

Long before a woman develops diabetes, insulin resistance is the predominant condition. Many women with PCOS have insulin resistance but have very normal blood sugar. Diabetes is insulin resistance taken one step further. After a meal, the blood sugar increases, and in an insulin-resistant person, a lot of insulin is needed to manage the sugar. The beta cells of the pancreas will struggle to make enough insulin and increase their output as much as possible. At some point, the beta cells are not able to manage the blood sugar any longer, and the blood sugar starts to rise higher than is optimal.

At this point, similar to the lipotoxicity we talked about earlier, glucolipotoxicity starts happening inside of the pancreas. It's a very long word meaning that there is a combination of high glucose and high free fatty acids that damage beta cells of the pancreas with inflammation.

This is an oversimplification, but a recent study found that removing one gram of fat directly from the pancreas was able to reverse type 2 diabetes.[1] This confirms the idea that free fatty acids and inflammatory cytokine mediators are involved in the damage to the beta cells. Once the beta cells are damaged, blood sugar becomes more and more out of control. This is diabetes.

Now you can see why women with PCOS are prone to diabetes, as both inflammation and insulin resistance are central in its development. Although the treatment of diabetes is out of the scope of this book, I hope you'll see that there is a lot that you can do to prevent it with the right nutrition and lifestyle.

Cardiovascular Disease

Having PCOS is linked with an increased risk of cardiovascular disease due to metabolic risks, high LDL and low HDL cholesterol, hypertension, and insulin resistance. Up to seventy percent of women in the United States with PCOS have been found to have high cholesterol, and a systematic review found that women with PCOS had double the risk for developing cardiovascular disease. This review also found that this risk was not completely related to higher body mass index. Even lean women had an increased risk.[2] Each and every one of us needs to pay attention to this risk.

It is important to note that the source of androgens may be associated with the degree of risk of cardiovascular disease. It appears that those who have predominantly high androgens from the adrenal glands, as evidenced by high DHEA-S levels, have a lower risk of cardiovascular disease when compared to those whose testosterone levels are more predominant. So, if you've had high testosterone, you may want to do more as you get older to keep your heart healthy.

Nonalcoholic Fatty Liver Disease

Nonalcoholic fatty liver disease (NAFLD) is a common condition found in women with PCOS. This is the most common liver disease worldwide, affecting a whopping twenty to thirty percent of people in the developed world. In NAFLD, fat is deposited into the liver cells, and the liver changes its structure and function as a result. The most concerning thing about NAFLD is that it is an independent risk factor for cardiovascular disease. Even if you have nothing else, NAFLD will put you at risk, so we need to identify and reverse it as soon as possible.

In chapter 3, we talked about how excess calories from fructose, glucose, and carbohydrates spill over and are stored in the liver cells. The liver can't process the food energy that it is presented with, which under normal circumstances, it would be able to process and eliminate.

To make matters worse, the fat stored in the liver undergoes lipotoxicity and oxidative stress. This can damage the liver cells. If NAFLD progresses long enough, this damage can become permanent, causing a condition known as nonalcoholic steatohepatitis (NASH). Fortunately, if you catch it quickly enough, NAFLD is completely reversible.

A study released in January 2013 in the *Journal of Human Reproductive Sciences* looked at a group of one hundred women, approximately half of whom had PCOS. It was determined that sixty-seven percent of women with PCOS had a fatty liver, compared to only twenty-five percent of the control group. We know that women with PCOS are at risk for this disease, and it has been suggested by some studies that high levels of androgens, which most women with PCOS have, are a risk factor that can lead to fatty liver.[3]

Reversing NAFLD

Following are some things you can do to start reversing NAFLD:

1. Aim to keep your waist circumference under thirty-five inches if you are of average frame. Small-framed women should aim for a waist circumference of less than thirty-two inches. This alone will significantly reduce your likelihood of having NAFLD. Abdominal circumference reflects abdominal fat deposition, much of which occurs around your liver.

2. Follow the recommendations in this book for diet and lifestyle. Minimizing insulin resistance is the key to reducing fatty liver.

3. Even a three to five percent weight loss can improve fatty liver, so focus on doing what you can gradually.

4. Eliminate sugars from your diet entirely. As the liver's fat deposits are

primarily made of triglycerides, sugar and refined carbs are quite simply the worst offenders in the list of causes for fatty liver.

5. Avoid excessive alcohol, which only worsens NAFLD, as it increases the fatty deposits and can produce inflammatory changes in the liver. Interestingly, light alcohol consumption may actually be helpful when it comes to combatting the illness: A study using the National Health and Nutrition data from 8,000 participants found that the consumption of one glass of wine per day cut the risk of NAFLD by half.[4]

6. Increase choline in your diet by consuming choline-rich foods. Choline has a special protective role in the liver in that it provides a way for the fat to be excreted through VLDL cholesterol. If there is a deficiency in choline, the liver will be less able to package up and excrete fats into the bloodstream. Rich sources of choline include egg yolks, organic grass-fed liver, and wild fish (as shown in Table C-1). The amount of choline required to treat fatty liver depends on diet: The richer one's diet is in refined foods, carbohydrates, and poor-quality oils, the more choline will be required. The recommended daily allowance (RDA) for choline is 500 mg, but in NAFLD the needs are likely much higher.

7. Avoid the consumption of refined, poor-quality vegetable oils. Consuming polyunsaturated vegetable oils when fatty liver is present will actually cause a quicker progression to the inflammatory NASH.[5] This is because these types of oils are quicker to oxidize and produce inflammation in the liver. Instead, choose high-quality, cold-pressed vegetable oils, such as extra virgin olive oil for low-heat cooking and extra virgin coconut oil for high-heat cooking, for more stability against oxidation.

8. Include a high-quality B vitamin supplement, including B12, B6, and folate. Eat spinach, which is a rich source of betaine. These nutrients will help spare choline in the body, helping the liver to excrete excess fat.

9. Take alpha-lipoic acid. In a new study on mice with choline deficiency-induced fatty liver, it was found that administering alpha-lipoic acid improved the health of the liver by increasing antioxidant status and reducing damage-causing inflammation. It also helped to reduce the peroxidation of fats in the liver.[6]

10. Take milk thistle. A 2012 randomized control trial on 179 patients with fatty liver disease found that milk thistle (also known as silymarin) improved liver enzymes, HOMA-IR, and produced a more normal cellular appearance of the liver.[7] Milk thistle can be taken as a tea, a capsule, or as a tincture.

Table C-1: Choline in Selected Foods

FOOD	MG OF CHOLINE PER 100MG SERVING
Egg-yolk	680
Egg-whole	270
Beef liver (pan-cooked)	430
Chicken liver	330
Pork-ham (lean)	110
Alaskan wild salmon	96
Cod	84
Flaxseeds	79
Amaranth	70
Quinoa	70
Almonds	52
Broccoli (cooked)	40
Brussel sprouts (cooked)	42
Pumpkin seeds	39
Kidney beans	33
Broccoli (raw)	19

Data taken from the USDA Database for Choline Content of Common Foods.

PCOS And Cancer

Many women with PCOS are concerned about cancer, in particular ovarian and breast cancer. Although it is a far more minimal risk compared to metabolic risks such as insulin resistance, type 2 diabetes, and cardiovascular disease, it is helpful to be aware of this, as the types of cancer in PCOS are among the most preventable.

The main cancer of concern is endometrial cancer. When cycles are long, estrogen has relatively longer periods of time to act on the endometrial lining, causing it to thicken. If ovulation doesn't happen, there is very little progesterone to change the structure of the lining and allow it to shed.

As such, some women with PCOS have a thickened endometrial lining, called endometrial hyperplasia. If this is allowed to go on unchecked, it is associated with an increased risk of endometrial cancer. A 2015 Danish study found that there was a fourfold increased risk of endometrial cancer in a group of 12,070 women with PCOS.[8] It's important not to panic, however, as the vast majority were type 1, which is low grade, slow spreading, and often treatable. It's also important to note that although there was a fourfold increase in endometrial cancer, only sixteen of the 12,070 women had it, as opposed to the typical statistics for endometrial cancer, where we would expect four women to be affected. This would mean that your chance of getting endometrial cancer would increase from 0.03 percent to 0.13 percent. Not a huge amount, but something to be aware of, as you can detect this early and treat it.

As such, for women who don't ovulate regularly, it is important to have a pelvic ultrasound and endometrial biopsy annually to check the health of the lining.

It is generally a good idea as well to induce a period every three months if you tend to go long periods of time without menses. An exception to this is after stopping birth control or having a baby. In these situations, it can take some time for things to kick back in for women with PCOS, and in many of these instances, estrogen levels are on the lower side. In any case, if you haven't had a period after six months of stopping the birth control pill, and you have PCOS, it's advisable to request an ultrasound and hormonal bloodwork, including LH, FSH, estradiol, and progesterone. This way, you can get an idea of how your ovaries and lining are doing.

The same Danish study also investigated other cancers and their link to PCOS. The study found no association between PCOS and breast or ovarian cancer, which is in line with the majority of evidence at this point. The study did find a minimal increase in ovarian cancer in younger women with PCOS, but the increase wasn't significant.

However, PCOS was associated with increased risks of colon, brain, and kidney cancers—a surprising finding for the researchers. In the end, they attributed the risks of both kidney and colon cancers primarily to increased body mass index and insulin resistance and not inherently to PCOS itself.

With respect to brain tumors, these were mostly located in the pituitary gland. This is in alignment with previous research associating benign microadenomas in the pituitary with PCOS. These growths can secrete prolactin and can cause hormonal imbalances, but they are almost always benign. It's been found that up to twenty-two percent of people have pituitary adenomas, and the vast majority are unaware of them.[9]

The bottom line is that you want to watch your endometrial lining carefully and be sure you don't go for long periods of time without periods. When it comes to other cancers, we can focus on the nutrition and lifestyle factors described in this book, and it's likely that these will reduce our risks, since most of them are metabolic in nature. And of course, environment is very important when it comes to any form of cancer, given that many environmental toxins that are problematic for PCOS can also contain risk for cancer. As an example, BPA can induce the growth of endometrial cancer cell lines and has been associated with ovarian and breast cancer risk.

Fortunately, if you are following the 8 steps, you'll already be taking the right precautions to protect yourself from cancer, cardiovascular disease, and type 2 diabetes. So, even if your periods become regular naturally as you get older, working on this program will help you to live a healthy, happy, and long life.

RECOMMENDED DIETS AND RECIPES FOR WOMEN WITH PCOS

Recipes and Sample 1 Week Meal Plan—Insulin Counting

In this appendix, I hope to provide you with a lot of ideas on how to make your nutrition plan work. I've included two main plans, with the option for a third with a little bit of modification. These are based on insulin counting and the 8 steps nutritional recommendations.

In addition to the plan outlined in this book, I have found that a variety of other nutrition plans can work well for women with PCOS. These include paleo, ketogenic, and carbohydrate counting, or glycemic load. First, I'll outline a couple of the most popular nutrition plans for PCOS before going into the 8 steps insulin-counting meal plan and recipes.

Paleo Diet

This is an excellent diet, as most meals are vegetable based, and it recommends high-quality animal protein sources such as grass-fed meats with plenty of healthful fats. The 8 steps insulin-counting program is very similar to paleo in that it is based on the consumption of whole foods, with plant foods as the center of the diet, and with avoidance of inflammatory foods like gluten and dairy.

The main difference in the insulin-counting program is that, for some women, portion-controlled rice and quinoa are occasionally included in the 8 steps program if the insulin count is kept in target range for that meal. I have found that rice is rather well tolerated by most women, and so there's no reason to be strict about excluding it completely. It also allows more flexibility with the menu by adding an enjoyable food that many cultures include as a staple. Another difference is that some women do really well with legumes, like lentils. I don't recommend eating legumes with every meal, due to their phytate content, but many women are able to consume them without any issue.

In addition, there are paleo "treats," which are popular within some circles. For women with PCOS, paleo treats are often not the best option, even though they are gluten free. They do contain sugars, and although the sugar choices made within the paleo diet are often optimal, the amount of sugar must be watched very closely for insulin resistant women. Occasionally, however, a treat may be enjoyed with a sweetener like stevia. I have included some of these in the plan.

As such, if you decide to follow a paleo diet, just be sure to keep paleo treats to a very occasional indulgence. Overall, the paleo diet works very well for many women with PCOS. It is easy to follow, and there are plenty of resources and supports available online.

Ketogenic Diet

This is a low-carbohydrate diet, which focuses on consuming a high proportion of dietary calories from fat and bringing net carbs to an absolute minimum, typically from thirty to fifty grams of net carbs per day. Net carbs are the total carbs you eat minus the fiber. (Fiber doesn't count!) Once the carbohydrate intake is very low, the body will shift into a different metabolic state, called ketosis. In ketosis, the brain uses the products of fat burning for fuel. The body shifts into fat metabolism, and many people lose significant amounts of weight. Although this diet has worked well for those who have larger amounts of weight to lose, it has its downfalls as well. For example, it may cause fatigue in some people, particularly those who are exercising. There is also little long-term research on this diet, except for patients with epilepsy. It is also associated with rapid weight loss and increases in cortisol, particularly if net carb consumption becomes very low. That being said, some women with PCOS have had wonderful success with this program, and with a doctor's supervision it can be safe and effective for some.

8 Steps Insulin-Counting Program

The insulin-counting program meal plan and recipes are good for women with all recommended insulin counts. Simply adjust the portion of what you eat to match the count you have determined is best for you in chapter 9. This plan follows everything you've learned in the nutrition chapter, giving you practical suggestions to make eating healthy easy and delicious! Many women who are insulin resistant do better without between meal snacks and others need them. In some cases, too much snacking, especially continuous grazing, can be a problem because insulin levels never really reduce to allow cells to become sensitive again.

For breakfast, many women do best keeping their insulin count below forty-five and adding more healthy fats, such as avocado, which provide metabolic benefits throughout the day.

Following the 1 week 8 Steps insulin counting meal plan, there is another option: the 8 Steps HFLC. Although similar to the ketogenic diet, the HFLC plan is not rigid on the absolute number of net carbs, but rather it is a variation of the first plan with a lower insulin count. You may find this optimal if you are striving for a lower insulin count plan due to significant insulin resistance. I usually recommend this program to women who have very insulin resistant metabolisms and, despite their best efforts on the regular insulin-counting program, are not able to lose weight.

This second, more intensive HFLC plan is best followed with a doctor's supervision, since it may require adjustments along the way. With respect to snacking, many women with significant insulin resistance do best avoiding it, increasing the amount of healthy fats with their meals, and fasting for fourteen hours after dinner until the next morning. That said, I've included some snack ideas because some women do not feel well without snacking. Always adjust to your individual needs, and drink plenty of fluids.

Lean PCOS and Nutrition

Lean and athletic women, take note. The vast majority of you will do better on the insulin-counting program and not on the HFLC plan, but with a much more flexible quantity of food and with the higher insulin counts recommended previously.

If you are lean or active, it's important to listen to your body, and not push too far trying to reduce insulin. Many lean women already have low-normal insulin, and so reducing it further can wreak havoc with your hormones. Focus instead on consuming the types of foods that you see here, and if you need more, then add what you need according to how you feel.

Athletes will have special needs for additional carbohydrates, particularly either before or after working out. These can fit very well into this program. Please consult with your trainer to determine your unique needs for the level of activity you're involved in.

Let's begin with the basic recipes for our two meal plans: insulin counting and 8 steps HFLC. After the recipes, a one-week meal plan will follow.

Breakfast

Blueberry Avocado Super Smoothie
Ingredients

> ½ avocado
>
> ½ cup ice
>
> 1 cup of frozen blueberries
>
> 1 tablespoon ground flax seeds
>
> 1 cup unsweetened almond milk
>
> 25 grams vegan protein powder
>
> ½ teaspoon cinnamon

Servings: 1

Approximate insulin count: 38

Coconut Chai Smoothie
Ingredients

> 1 cup unsweetened coconut or almond milk
>
> ½ cup ice
>
> 1 teaspoon vanilla extract
>
> 1 teaspoon ginger
>
> 1 teaspoon cinnamon
>
> A pinch of allspice
>
> 2 tablespoons macadamia nut butter
>
> ¼ cup shredded coconut
>
> 25 grams vegan protein powder
>
> 1 tablespoon chia seed

Servings: 1

Approximate insulin count: 44

Egg Muffins with Prosciutto

Ingredients

> 12 eggs
>
> 10 slices of prosciutto, chopped
>
> 2 red peppers, finely chopped
>
> 1 large onion, finely chopped
>
> 4 cups chopped baby spinach
>
> ½ teaspoon salt
>
> ½ teaspoon black pepper
>
> 2 tablespoons avocado oil plus extra for greasing the muffin tins

Instructions

- Preheat oven to 375 degrees. Grease the tins with avocado oil. Heat two teaspoons of avocado oil in a skillet over low-medium heat.
- Cook red peppers and onions until they start to soften, then add chopped spinach and prosciutto, and cook until the spinach has just wilted.
- Whisk the eggs in a bowl, then season with salt and pepper. Add veggie mixture with prosciutto and combine. Scoop the egg and veggie/prosciutto mixture into the greased muffin tins.
- Bake the muffins at 375 degrees for twenty minutes, or until cooked. After cooling, remove from muffin tins and store in the fridge to be used for breakfast on the go!

Servings: 4 (3 muffins per serving)

Approximate insulin count: 29

Greens and Berries Cashew Smoothie

Ingredients

> 1 cup frozen raspberries or blackberries
>
> ½ cup ice
>
> 1 cup spinach leaves
>
> 1 cup unsweetened vanilla almond milk
>
> 1 tablespoon cashew butter
>
> 25 grams vegan protein powder

Servings: 1

Approximate insulin count: 37

Omelet with Mushrooms and Spinach
Ingredients
¼ medium onion

1 tablespoon avocado oil

2 heaping cups of spinach

1 cup of sliced mushrooms

3 eggs

2 tablespoons canned coconut milk (LCHF version only)

1 medium spring onion (garnish)

1 medium chopped tomato

Salt and pepper to taste

Instructions
- Slice onion into long strips and then sauté them in oil until caramelized. Add spinach to the pan and allow it to wilt. Remove vegetables from the pan. Mix three large eggs, coconut milk, and salt and pepper together in a container.
- Pour egg mixture into the pan and allow it to cook over medium-low heat. Once edges of omelet begin to set, spoon spinach and onions over half of the omelet. As the top of the omelet begins to set, fold over the omelet and serve! Garnish with spring onions if you'd like.

Servings: 1

Approximate insulin count: 24

Protein Pancakes
Ingredients
1 banana, mashed

2 eggs, whisked

2 tablespoons coconut flour

¼ cup unsweetened almond milk

1 scoop unsweetened vegan protein powder

Avocado oil

(A spray bottle is convenient for pancakes.)

Instructions
- Combine the banana, eggs, and almond milk in a bowl. Mix dry ingredients in another bowl.
- Add the wet ingredients into the dry ingredients and stir until they are combined thoroughly.
- Spray a medium skillet or pancake grill with avocado oil spray. Over low-medium

heat, add pancake batter to the skillet. Cook as you would typical pancakes, watching carefully to ensure they are not burning.

- Top with fresh blackberries or raspberries and cinnamon if desired and enjoy!

Servings: 2

Approximate insulin count: 36 plus toppings

Sunshine Kale Breakfast Hash

Ingredients

    2 cups kale, sliced

    1 clove garlic, minced

    ½ teaspoon sea salt

    Freshly ground pepper to taste

    1 small roasted sweet potato cut in small cubes (Tip: roast some for the week and store in the fridge, or purchase frozen diced sweet potato cubes for busy mornings.) Substitute zucchini for 8 steps HFLC.

    2 large eggs

    1 tablespoon avocado oil plus 1 tablespoon for 8 steps HFLC

Instructions

- In a skillet on medium heat, add one-half tablespoon of the avocado oil. Add kale, minced garlic, sea salt, pepper, and one tablespoon of water.
- Cook until the kale has wilted and the garlic is fragrant, about two minutes.
- Add the roasted sweet potatoes (or zucchini) and sauté gently for about about two minutes (five minutes for zucchini).
- When everything is hot, place the veggies on a plate and cover to keep them warm. Add the other ½ tablespoon avocado oil to the skillet, and cook the eggs as you like them (over-easy is often delicious with this recipe). Add salt and pepper to taste.
- Place the eggs on top of the veggie hash and enjoy!

Servings: 2

Approximate insulin count: 26

Snacks

Chia Pudding
Ingredients
> ¼ cup chia seeds, whole or ground
>
> ¼ cup canned organic coconut milk
>
> ½ cup unsweetened almond milk
>
> 1 tablespoon raw cacao powder, unsweetened
>
> 5–10 drops liquid stevia extract
>
> ½ tablespoon raw cocoa nibs or extra dark chocolate (at least 85% cocoa solids)

Instructions
- Mix together (or blend for a smoother option) the chia seeds, coconut milk, water, cacao powder, and stevia. Put it in the fridge overnight to set. Top with raw cocoa nibs or dark chocolate. You can also make it fresh, but you'll need to let it set for around ten minutes before eating. Makes one serving.

Servings: 1

Approximate insulin count: 7

Choco-Blueberry Almond "Cereal"
Ingredients
> ½ cup of blueberries
>
> 1 cup of unsweetened coconut milk (carton, not can)
>
> 2 tablespoons almonds, slivered
>
> ½ tablespoon raw cacao powder

Instructions
- Place into a bowl for a super-fast snack and enjoy!

Servings: 1

Approximate insulin count: 3

Granola Chocolate Nut Bars
Ingredients

> 1 cup almonds
>
> 1 cup sunflower seeds
>
> ½ cup macadamia nuts
>
> 1 cup unsweetened coconut flakes
>
> 1 egg
>
> ¼ cup coconut butter (available at a health food store)
>
> ¼ cup almond butter
>
> ½ cup dark chocolate chips
>
> 2 tablespoons vanilla extract
>
> ½ teaspoon cinnamon

Instructions

- Preheat the oven to 350 degrees and rub a shallow glass baking dish with coconut oil. Place all of the ingredients into a blender and then blend coarsely. Pour all ingredients into the pan and press them out evenly.
- Bake for about thirteen to fifteen minutes. Cut into sixteen pieces. You can freeze batches of this, so you have easy snacks on the go.

Servings: 16

Approximate insulin count: 10

Guacamole
Ingredients

> 4 fresh avocados, pitted and mashed
>
> 2 Roma tomatoes, chopped
>
> 1 garlic clove, pressed
>
> Juice of two limes
>
> ¼ teaspoon cumin
>
> ¼ teaspoon chili powder
>
> ½ teaspoon sea salt
>
> Fresh ground black pepper, to taste
>
> 2 tablespoons fresh cilantro, finely chopped

Instructions

- Mash the avocado in a bowl, then pour the lime juice over the avocado right away. This will stop it from turning brown. Mix in the tomatoes and the rest of the spices, and you're done!

Servings: 7

Approximate insulin count: 4

Protein-Packed Apple Cinnamon Muffins

Ingredients

    5 eggs

    1 cup unsweetened applesauce

    ½ cup coconut flour

    2 tablespoons cinnamon

    1 teaspoon baking soda

    1 teaspoon vanilla

    ¼ cup coconut oil

Instructions

- Preheat the oven to 400 degrees. Grease your muffin tin lightly with coconut oil. Whisk all of the ingredients together in a large bowl, then let them sit for around five minutes. Place about one-third cup of batter in each muffin tin.
- Bake until they begin to brown, about eleven to fifteen minutes. They should not be soft when lightly touched on the top. Let them cool. Muffins may be frozen or refrigerated for a quick breakfast on the go on a busy morning.

Servings: 12

Approximate insulin count: 8

Zucchini Crisps with Lemon Thyme

Ingredients

    1 medium zucchini

    Juice of ½ lemon, squeezed

    ½ teaspoon sea salt

    2 teaspoons olive oil

    1 teaspoon thyme

    ¼ teaspoon ground pepper

Instructions

- Slice zucchini into one-fourth-inch circles. Sprinkle zucchini with salt and lemon juice and place on a colander to drain.
- Preheat oven to 250 degrees and line a baking sheet with parchment paper. Brush parchment with one teaspoon of oil. Pat zucchini slices dry with a paper towel and arrange them on the baking sheet. Brush the tops with the remaining oil and sprinkle with thyme, salt, and ground pepper.
- Bake forty-five minutes, watching to ensure they don't overcook. Then, turn off oven and let chips sit in the oven for around an hour, until they become crisp. Serves two.

Servings: 2

Approximate insulin count: 3

Lunch

Cashew Mustard Turkey Wrap
Ingredients

    4 ounces all-natural deli or roasted turkey

    1 large lettuce leaf (butter lettuce or collard greens are best)

    5 grape tomatoes, halved lengthways

    1 tablespoon purple onion (thinly sliced)

    ¼ red or yellow bell pepper

    1 tablespoon mustard

    1 tablespoon cashew butter

Instructions

- Wash and dry your lettuce or collard. Spread mustard and cashew butter on the leaf.
- Place the onion, bell pepper, and the grape tomatoes on top. Roll and pin securely with toothpicks to keep the wrap together. Cut in half and enjoy. Serves one.

Servings: 1

Approximate insulin count: 16

Curried Chicken Salad with Apples
Ingredients

    1 small Gala apple, peeled, cored, and diced (omit apple for 8 steps HFLC)

    ½ pound cooked chicken breast or thighs

    ¼ cup homemade mayo or all-natural mayo

    1 cup chopped celery

    2 spring onions (scallions), white and green parts, chopped

    ¾ teaspoon curry powder

    1 teaspoon sea salt

    Freshly ground black pepper to taste

    ½ lemon, juiced

    ½ cup parsley, chopped

    ¼ cup cashews

Instructions

- Mix the mayonnaise and curry powder in a bowl, and then add salt and pepper to taste. In a separate bowl, add the apple chunks and gently toss with the lemon juice. Shred or chop the chicken and add it to the apple/lemon mixture Fold in the green onions and mayonnaise until well combined and then enjoy!

Servings: 2

Approximate insulin count: 29.5

Hearty Chicken and Butternut Squash Soup

Ingredients

    4 bone-in, skinless chicken thighs
    ½ medium butternut squash (about 1 pound), peeled, seeded,
        and diced medium
    1 small yellow onion, diced medium
    2 tablespoons organic coconut oil
    Sea salt and pepper to taste
    4 cups homemade chicken bone broth, or organic chicken broth
    ¼ teaspoon ground cumin
    ½ teaspoon dried oregano
    2 tablespoons fresh lemon juice

Instructions

- Preheat oven to 425 degrees. Toss together chicken, squash, onion, and coconut oil. Season with salt and pepper, distributing evenly. Roast until both chicken and squash are cooked and tender, about thirty minutes.
- Transfer chicken to a plate and set aside. Add the cooked squash and onions to a medium pot, and then add broth, cumin, and oregano. Bring to a simmer over medium-high.
- With a potato masher, smash some of the vegetables (about half) to thicken the soup texture. Remove the skin and bones from chicken, cut it into small pieces, and add it to the soup. Add lemon juice and salt and pepper to taste. Enjoy.

Servings: 3

Approximate insulin count: 61

Salad in a Jar Options:

Olive Shrimp-Cobb Salad

Ingredients

2 tablespoons vinaigrette or creamy ranch dressing
2 tablespoons chopped avocado
8 grape tomatoes
1 tablespoon red onion, chopped
½ cup large chunks of cucumber
1 cup chopped romaine lettuce
8 black olives, sliced
8 cooked shrimp
1 boiled egg, quartered

Instructions
- In a large mason jar (or any other jar will work as well) layer the ingredients. Put the dressing on the bottom of the jar. Add the tomatoes, onions, and cucumber. Add the olives and avocado. Add the eggs and shrimp. The lettuce should be the top layer.
- When you are ready to eat, empty the jar into a bowl, mix, and enjoy!

Servings: 1

Approximate insulin count: 20

Raspberry Clementine Protein Salad
Ingredients

    2 tablespoons balsamic vinaigrette dressing

    ½ cup shredded carrots

    ¼ cup thinly sliced red onion

    ½ cup cherry tomatoes

    1 small clementine orange, sectioned

    ½ cup of raspberries

    2 hard-boiled eggs, sliced in half lengthways

    1 tablespoon sunflower seeds

    2 cups spring green mix

Instructions
- In a mason jar (or any other jar will work as well), layer the ingredients. Put the balsamic vinaigrette on the bottom of the jar. Add carrots, onion, and cherry tomatoes. Add clementine and raspberries. Add sunflower seeds and hard-boiled eggs. Add spring mix as the top layer of the jar. When you are ready to eat, empty the jar into a bowl, mix and enjoy!

Servings: 1

Approximate insulin count: 27

Wild Salmon Avocado Salad
Ingredients

    130 g canned or fresh wild salmon, well drained (canned salmon is usually wild)

    1–2 cups crispy romaine lettuce

    ½ carrot, diced

    ½ small red pepper, diced

    ½ cucumber, cubed

    ½ cup whole cherry tomatoes

    2 tablespoons chopped green onion

    ¼ avocado, sliced

    2 tablespoons creamy avocado ranch dressing

Instructions

- Layer the ingredients in a mason jar (or any other jar will work as well). Put the creamy avocado ranch dressing and then the salmon on the bottom of the jar. Add carrots, red peppers, tomato, onion, avocado, and green onion. Add romaine as the top layer of the jar. When ready to eat, empty the jar into a bowl, mix and enjoy!

Servings: 1

Approximate insulin count: 31

Skewered Chicken Kebabs
Ingredients

    4 ounces leftover roast chicken (or another leftover meat)

    ½ cucumber, cut into large chunks

    ½ cup red pepper, cut into large chunks

    ½ medium zucchini, cut into chunks

Instructions

- Place the ingredients on two skewers for a quick lunch. Enjoy with two tablespoons of either mayo or creamy avocado ranch dressing!

Servings: 1

Approximate insulin count: 23

Spicy Chicken Crock-Pot Soup

Ingredients

    3 medium boneless chicken thighs

    1 teaspoon onion powder

    1 teaspoon garlic powder

    ½ teaspoon dried celery seed

    ¼ cup avocado oil

    ½–3 teaspoons chili flakes, depending on how spicy you want it!

    3 cups beef bone broth or organic boxed beef broth

    1 cup canned coconut milk

    ¼ teaspoon tapioca starch

    Salt and pepper to taste

Instructions

- Cut the chicken into chunks, and add it to the Crock-Pot with onion and garlic powder, celery seed, avocado oil, broth, and chili flakes.
- Put the Crock-Pot on low heat for six hours and let everything cook completely. Once everything is cooked, remove the chicken from the Crock-Pot and roughly shred it by pulling it apart with a fork. Add the coconut milk and tapioca starch to the Crock-Pot.
- Use an immersion blender to emulsify all of the liquids together in the Crock-Pot, or blend everything (less the chicken) in a blender then place it back in the pot afterward.
- Place the pulled chicken back into the Crock-Pot and stir. Season to taste. Serves five.

Servings: 5

Approximate insulin count: 23

Creamy Broccoli Slaw

Ingredients

> 2 ½ cups of organic broccoli slaw (you can find this in the cooler in the
> vegetable section)
>
> 1 small tomato, chopped
>
> 1 avocado, cubed
>
> 1 small zucchini, chopped
>
> 2 tablespoons balsamic vinaigrette dressing

Instructions

- Place the broccoli slaw, avocado, tomato, and zucchini in a large bowl, and gently combine. Add balsamic vinaigrette dressing. Toss to combine. Season with salt and pepper to taste. Enjoy!

Servings: 2

Approximate insulin count: 4

Dinner

Asian Garlicky Ginger Chicken
Ingredients

>4 bone-in, skin-on chicken thighs, organic or pastured (if not available, get skinless)
>
>½ tablespoon coconut oil
>
>Sea salt and black pepper to taste
>
>1 small onion, sliced
>
>1 teaspoon sesame seeds
>
>1–2 pinches chili flakes, depending on your heat preference
>
>2 cloves of garlic, chopped (or 1 teaspoon garlic powder)
>
>½ teaspoon ginger, powder or fresh
>
>1 tablespoon unsweetened rice vinegar
>
>¼ cup coconut aminos (soy sauce substitute at health food stores)

Instructions
- Preheat the oven to 425 degrees. Lightly season the chicken on both sides with salt and pepper.
- Melt the coconut oil in a skillet on medium heat, then add the chicken to the pan, skin side down, and cook until it browns. (If you are using a skinless variety, you will need to use more coconut oil.)
- As the chicken is browning in the skillet, combine the onion, garlic, ginger, sesame seeds, chili flakes, coconut aminos, rice vinegar, and more sea salt and black pepper in a small mixing bowl. Turn the chicken skin-side up in the pan, and cover it with the sauce.
- Put the pan into the oven for thirty minutes if you are using stainless steel or cast iron. If not, transfer it to a glass baking pan. Ensure the chicken is thoroughly cooked, and enjoy!

Servings: 2

Approximate insulin count: 51

Chicken Cacciatore over "Spaghetti"

Ingredients

    4–6 pieces of skinless chicken (legs or breasts)
    1 medium spaghetti squash
    1 teaspoon (4 grams) Celtic sea salt
    Black pepper to taste
    2 tablespoons avocado oil
    1 chopped onion
    1 large chopped red pepper
    2 cloves chopped garlic
    1 can diced organic tomatoes (with juice, nothing else added)
    1 cup water
    1 bay leaf
    1 teaspoon oregano
    1 teaspoon basil
    Hot pepper flakes, if desired

Instructions

- Rinse the chicken, then pat dry. Sprinkle with ½ teaspoon of salt and pepper.
- Preheat oven to 400 degrees. Slice the spaghetti squash lengthwise, and place it face down on a baking sheet. Bake for thirty-five to forty minutes, until the threads can be easily removed from the squash with a fork.
- Heat a large pan over medium-low heat. Add two tablespoons of avocado oil to warm slightly. Add garlic and onions and sauté for one minute.
- Add chicken and cook until brown on one side, flip over and brown the other side. Add the peppers, tomatoes, water, bay leaf, oregano, basil, hot pepper flakes, and one-half teaspoon of salt; bring to a simmer. Cover and simmer until sauce has thickened, about twenty-five minutes.
- Add in spaghetti squash threads and mix until well combined. Turn heat to low and let simmer for about ten minutes, until chicken is tender. Add salt and pepper to taste. Garnish with parsley and black pepper. Serve with two cups steamed broccoli drizzled with one tablespoon of extra virgin olive oil.

Servings: 4

Approximate insulin count: 55

Crock Pot Comfort Roast Beef

Ingredients

   1 grass-fed chuck roast

   3.5 cups homemade beef bone broth (or 1 900 ml carton all natural
       organic beef broth

   5 carrots, cut into chunks

   1 onion, chopped

   3 cloves of garlic, smashed

   2 stalks of celery, cut into chunks

   3 pieces of rosemary, leaves removed from stem

   Salt and pepper to taste

   Chopped parsley or green onion to garnish

Instructions

- Generously sprinkle all sides of the roast with salt and pepper. Heat avocado oil
  in a pan, then sear all sides of the roast for five to six minutes each. Combine all
  ingredients in your Crock-Pot and then cook on low for eight to ten hours.

Servings: 5

Approximate insulin count: 51

Bone Broth

Ingredients

> Bone (of entire organic, pastured chicken, or 3–4 pounds of grass-fed beef bone)
> 3 cups of roughly chopped vegetables, including carrots, celery, and a leafy green such as spinach
> 2 onions
> 6 smashed garlic cloves
> Celtic or Himalayan sea salt to taste
> 1 tablespoon apple cider vinegar
> Water to fill Crock-Pot
> Herbs to taste including 1 bay leaf, 1 sprig of thyme or rosemary

Instructions

- Place the vegetables into a large slow cooker. Place the bones on top of the vegetables. Pour the vinegar on top of the bones, and then sprinkle salt and the herbs on top. Turn on the slow cooker and cook on low for ten to fifteen hours.
- Pour the broth through a strainer and discard or compost the solids. Pour it into a large container and refrigerate overnight.
- The fat will solidify on the top. Skim this layer off and discard. The broth may look gelatinous but that is normal. Heat and enjoy!
- Store leftover bone broth for a couple of days in the refrigerator or ladle out into mason jars and freeze. If you are using mason jars, be sure to leave lots of extra space on top, so that the jar doesn't break when the broth freezes!

    Note: If you don't have a slow cooker, you can still make bone broth. Use a large pot, and cook on low for ten hours. You'll have to stir occasionally and top up with water when needed.

    Insulin count for bone broth is zero.

Mediterranean Shrimp with Zucchini Noodles

Ingredients

- ½ cup shrimp, peeled and deveined
- 1 medium zucchini, julienned very slim like spaghetti (or use a spiralizer to make zucchini noodles)
- 1 onion, chopped
- 2 cloves garlic, chopped
- 1 can diced tomatoes, with liquid (14 ounces)
- 3 tablespoons black olives
- ½ can artichoke hearts (14 ounces), optional
- 2 cups fresh spinach
- ½ teaspoon red chili flakes
- 1 teaspoon fresh oregano
- 1 tablespoon fresh lemon juice
- 1 tablespoon coconut oil

Instructions

- Heat coconut oil in a large pan over medium heat until melted. Add onion and garlic and cook until the onion is transparent and the garlic is fragrant. Add the chili. Add artichokes and olives and cook for two to three minutes. Add the oregano and diced tomatoes and stir. Bring to a simmer. Cover and let simmer for ten minutes.
- Uncover, add zucchini and lemon juice, then cook, stirring continuously for about five minutes. Add shrimp. When the shrimp is just cooked through, add the spinach.
- Add fresh lemon juice and salt and pepper to taste. Serve and enjoy!

Servings: 1

Approximate insulin count: 25

Mushroom Sausage Pizza Spaghetti Bake

Ingredients

   1 large spaghetti squash

   1 pound no-sugar-added, all-natural chicken sausage

   ½ onion, chopped

   1 cup button mushrooms, chopped

   1 cup pizza sauce (no sugar added)

   1 teaspoon dried basil

   1 teaspoon dried oregano

   Salt and pepper to taste

   3 eggs, whisked

Instructions

- Preheat the oven to 400 degrees. Grease an eight-by-eight baking dish with coconut oil. Cut spaghetti squash in half lengthwise. Place spaghetti squash cut side down on a baking sheet and bake for twenty to twenty-five minutes. Reduce the oven temperature to 350 degrees.
- Remove the threads from the spaghetti squash and spread them out evenly in the dish. Warm up a pan on medium heat. Add the sausage, mushrooms, and onion. Sauté sausage until it is cooked through and the onion is tender.
- Add the pizza sauce, oregano, basil, and salt and pepper to the pan and mix well. Add sausage mixture to dish and mix it with the spaghetti squash so it is distributed evenly. Add the whisked eggs to the dish and mix everything thoroughly.
- Bake for one hour, or until a crust has formed on top of the bake. Let sit for five minutes. Cut, serve, and enjoy!

Servings: 4

Approximate insulin count: 64

Pan-Seared Salmon with Dill Dressing

Ingredients

> Wild salmon fillet with skin on
> 2 tablespoons avocado oil
> Sea salt and black pepper to taste
> Creamy avocado ranch dressing (found in sauces section)

Instructions

- Pat the salmon dry, then season it with salt and pepper. Heat one tablespoon of avocado oil in a skillet over medium-high heat.
- Place the salmon, with skin facing down, in the skillet and then turn down the heat to medium-low. Gently press each piece of salmon down with a spatula, so that they crisp and stay nice and flat. Cook for six to seven minutes.
- Sear the other sides of the salmon for thirty seconds per side. Ensure that it is cooked (it should flake with a fork). Place the salmon on a plate and serve with creamy avocado ranch dressing.

Servings: 1

Approximate insulin count: 34

Simple Mashed Garlicky Cauliflower

Ingredients

> 3 cloves of garlic, smashed
> 1 large cauliflower head, broken into big chunks
> 1 tablespoon minced rosemary
> 1 tablespoon extra virgin olive oil
> Salt and pepper to taste

Instructions

- Smash a few cloves of garlic into one-fourth cup of olive oil. Let it infuse for at least a few minutes, then remove garlic pieces. Bring a large pot of water to a boil, then add a small handful of sea salt. Add the cauliflower and simmer until it is tender, usually from twelve to fifteen minutes.
- Blend the cauliflower in a food processor with three-fourths of the garlic, olive oil, rosemary, and a few generous pinches of salt and pepper. Adjust flavoring by tasting and adding salt, pepper, or more rosemary. Add the last of the olive oil. Serve and enjoy!

Servings: 2

Approximate insulin count: 22

Southwest Turkey Taco Salad

Ingredients

　　6 cups romaine lettuce, chopped

　　2 large tomatoes, diced

　　1 avocado, cubed

　　¼ red onion, slivered

　　1 small bunch cilantro leaves

　　2 limes, quartered

　　2 tablespoons avocado oil

　　2 pounds ground turkey

　　1 onion, chopped

　　2 garlic cloves, minced

　　1 teaspoon cumin

　　2 tablespoons chili powder

　　1 small pinch cinnamon

　　Salt and pepper to taste

　　Coconut oil for cooking

Instructions

- Place romaine, tomatoes, avocados, red onion, and cilantro leaves in a large bowl, then drizzle them with olive oil and lightly toss.
- Heat one tablespoon coconut oil in a pan. Add onion and sauté until transparent. Add garlic, spices, and one teaspoon of salt and sauté for one minute. Stir in the ground turkey, and brown it for five to ten minutes.
- Pour the taco meat onto the salad, then squeeze the limes over the salad. Season with salt and pepper.

Servings: 3

Approximate insulin count: 3

Stir Fried Garlic Bok Choy

Ingredients

    ⅓ cup bone broth (chicken or beef)

    1 tablespoon coconut aminos

    1 ½ teaspoons tapioca starch

    3 tablespoons avocado oil

    4 cloves sliced garlic

    2 pounds baby or Shanghai bok choy, halved lengthwise

Instructions

- Stir together broth, coconut aminos, tapioca starch, and ½ teaspoon salt until tapioca starch has dissolved. Heat wok over medium heat. Coat wok with avocado oil.
- Add garlic and stir-fry briefly for ten seconds. Add half of bok choy and stir-fry until leaves wilt, then add remaining bok choy and stir-fry until all leaves are bright green and wilted, two to three minutes total.
- Stir broth mixture, then pour into wok and stir-fry for fifteen seconds. Cover with lid and allow the bok choy to cook until tender, stirring occasionally. Enjoy!

Servings: 2

Approximate insulin count: 4

Sauces and Condiments

These can be used on salads or as toppings or sauces for various dishes.

Balsamic Vinaigrette

Ingredients

    ¼ cup balsamic vinegar

    1 tablespoon chopped garlic

    1 teaspoon mustard powder

    ¾ cup extra virgin olive oil

    Salt and pepper to taste

Instructions

- Add to a glass jar and shake.

Servings: 6

Approximate insulin count: 3

Creamy Avocado Ranch Dressing
Ingredients
- 1 cup homemade mayonnaise
- ⅓ cup unsweetened almond milk
- ½ medium sized avocado (pitted and skinned)
- 1 clove of garlic
- ½ teaspoon dried chives
- ½ teaspoon dried parsley
- ½ teaspoon dried dill
- ¼ teaspoon onion powder
- ⅛ teaspoon Celtic sea salt
- ⅛ teaspoon black pepper

Instructions
- Blend all ingredients on low until combined and creamy. Taste and season with salt and pepper, if needed. Store in refrigerator.

Servings: 4
Approximate insulin count: 11

Homemade Mayonnaise
Ingredients
- 1 ¼ cups light olive oil, divided
- 1 egg, room temperature
- ½ cup fresh, room temperature lemon juice
- ½ teaspoon mustard powder
- ½ teaspoon fine ground sea salt or more to taste

Instructions
- Place the room temperature egg, one-fourth cup of the olive oil, mustard powder, and salt in a blender or food processor. Mix thoroughly. Process on low and gradually add remaining olive oil in a very slow, thin stream. After the mixture has emulsified, turn the blender off. With a spoon, gently stir in lemon juice to taste. Store in refrigerator.

Servings: 5
Approximate insulin count: 7

Insulin Counting One-Week Plan

Table D-1: One-Week Meal Plan

MEAL	DAY 1	DAY 2	DAY 3	DAY 4	DAY 5	DAY 6	DAY 7
Breakfast	3 Egg Muffins with Prosciutto	Blueberry Avocado Super Smoothie	3 Egg Muffins with Prosciutto	Protein Pancakes 2 tbsp almond butter and handful of raspberries	Coconut Chai Smoothie	Sunshine Kale Breakfast Hash	Omelet with Mushrooms and Spinach ½ orange on the side
Snack	Choco-Blueberry Almond "Cereal"	1/2 apple with 1 tbsp almond butter	Veggie sticks with 2 tbsp guacamole	½ cup of blueberries with 2 brazil nuts	1 Protein Packed Apple Cinnamon Muffin	Veggie sticks with 2 tbsp guacamole	½ medium orange with 2 brazil nuts
Lunch	Cashew Mustard Turkey Wrap	Wild Salmon Avocado Salad	Garlicky Chicken Skewers with veggies	Hearty Chicken and Butternut Squash Soup (made ahead, frozen) with Creamy Broccoli Slaw	Raspberry Clementine Protein Salad	Hearty Chicken and Butternut Squash Soup with steamed green beans	Curried Chicken Salad with apples
Snack	Veggie sticks with 3 tbsp guacamole	Chia Pudding	1 Protein Packed Apple Cinnamon Muffin	Choco-Blueberry Almond "Cereal"	1 Protein Packed Apple Cinnamon Muffin	Chia Pudding	1 Protein Packed Apple Cinnamon Muffin
Dinner	Pan-seared Salmon with Dill Dressing 2 cups steamed broccoli	Asian Garlicky Ginger Chicken Stir-Fried Garlic Bok Choy	Southwest Turkey Taco Salad	Mediterranean shrimp with zucchini noodles	Chicken Cacciatore over "Spaghetti"	Crock Pot Comfort Roast Beef Simple Mashed Garlicky Cauliflower	Mushroom Sausage Pizza Spaghetti Bake with garden salad and 1 tbsp vinaigrette dressing
Time Saving Options for Next Day	Prep extra salmon for salad tomorrow. Or, use canned salmon	Use leftover chicken to prepare skewers for lunch	Defrost Soup (premade) and prep Broccoli Slaw	Hard boil eggs and prep salad for lunch			

8 Steps HFLC One-Week Plan

Table D-2: One-Week Meal Plan

MEAL	DAY 1	DAY 2	DAY 3	DAY 4	DAY 5	DAY 6	DAY 7
Breakfast	3 Egg Muffins with Prosciutto	Chocolate Strawberry Smoothie	3 Egg Muffins with Prosciutto	Chia Pudding	Coconut Chai Smoothie	Sunshine Kale Breakfast Hash	Omelet with Mushrooms and Spinach
Snack	Celery sticks with 2 tbsp almond butter	Veggie sticks with 2 tbsp guacamole	Celery sticks with Almond Butter	Veggie sticks with 2 tbsp guacamole	Celery sticks with almond butter	Veggie sticks with 2 tbsp guacamole	Zucchini Crisps with guacamole
Lunch	Cashew Mustard Turkey Wrap	Wild Salmon Avocado Salad	Garlicky Chicken Skewers with veggies	Spicy Chicken Crock-Pot Soup / Creamy Broccoli Slaw	Olive Shrimp Cobb Salad	Spicy Chicken Crock-Pot Soup with steamed green beans	Curried Chicken Salad
Snack	1 Granola Choco Nut Protein Bar	Romaine lettuce rolled with 1 tbsp mayo and 1 turkey slice	1 Granola Choco Nut Protein Bar	1 boiled egg	1 Granola Choco Nut Protein Bar	Romaine lettuce rolled with 1 tbsp mayo and 1 turkey slice	1 Granola Choco Nut Protein Bar
Dinner	Pan seared Salmon with Dill Dressing / 2 cups steamed broccoli	Asian Garlicky Ginger Chicken / Stir Fried Garlic Bok Choy	Southwest Turkey Taco Salad	Mediterranean shrimp with Zucchini noodles	Chicken Cacciatore over "Spaghetti"	Crock-Pot Comfort Roast Beef / Simple Mashed Garlicky Cauliflower	Mushroom Sausage Pizza Spaghetti Bake / With Garden Salad and 1 tbsp balsamic vinaigrette
Time Saving Options for Next Day	Prep extra salmon for salad tomorrow. Or, use canned salmon	Use leftover chicken to prepare skewers for lunch	Defrost soup (pre-made) and prep Broccoli Slaw	Hard boil eggs and prep extra shrimp for lunch			

Books

- *A Patient's Guide to PCOS: Understanding—and Reversing—Polycystic Ovary Syndrome* by Dr. Walter Futterweit
- *The Infertility Cure* by Dr. Randine Lewis
- *Beat Diabetes Naturally* by Dr. Michael Murray
- *Period Repair Manual: Natural Treatment for Better Hormones and Better Periods* by Dr. Lara Briden
- *Taking Charge of Your Fertility: The Definitive Guide to Natural Birth Control, Pregnancy Achievement, and Reproductive Health* by Toni Weschler
- *The Adrenal Reset Diet: Strategically Cycle Carbs and Proteins to Lose Weight, Balance Hormones, and Move from Stressed to Thriving* by Dr. Alan Christianson
- *The Natural Diet Solution for PCOS and Infertility* by Dr. Nancy Dunne and Bill Slater
- *The New Glucose Revolution: Low GI Eating Made Easy* by Dr. Jennie Brand-Miller and Kaye Foster-Powell
- *The Obesity Code: Unlocking the Secrets of Weight Loss* by Dr. Jason Fung
- *The PCOS Workbook: Your Guide to Complete Physical and Emotional Health* by Angela Grassi
- *Woman Code: Perfect Your Cycle, Amplify Your Fertility, Supercharge Your Sex Drive, and Become a Power Source* by Alisa Vitti
- *Your Healthy Pregnancy with Thyroid Disease: A Guide to Fertility, Pregnancy, and Postpartum Wellness* by Mary Shomon and Dana Trentini. (Featuring contributions by Dr. Fiona McCulloch)
- *Women's Encyclopedia of Natural Medicine* by Dr. Tori Hudson

Labwork

Hormone and metabolic testing can be done at most major labs with a physician's requisition such as—

- Labcorp
- Lifelabs/CML and Gamma Dynacare (Canada)

Cortisol and Blood Hormonal Testing

- Cell Science Systems https://cellsciencesystems.com/
  - Adrenal Stress Profile
- Diagnostechs http://www.diagnostechs.com/
  - Adrenal Stress Index
- Genova Diagnostics http://gdx.net
  - Adrenocortex Stress Profile
- RMA Labs http://rmalab.com
  - Adrenal Function Panel
- ZRT Labs http://www.zrtlab.com/
  - Adrenal Stress Profile
  - Cardiometabolic Profile

Environmental Toxicity Testing

- Genova Diagnostics http://www.gdx.net
  - Toxic Effects
- Great Plains Labs http://www.greatplainslaboratory.com/
  - Toxic organic chemical Panel

MTHFR Testing

- 23andMe https://www.23andme.com/
- Cell Science Systems https://cellsciencesystems.com/
- Spectracell http://www.spectracell.com/

Specialized Metabolic Testing

- Genova Diagnostics http://gdx.net
  - Oxidative Stress 2.0 (includes lipid peroxides)
- Great Plains Labs http://www.greatplainslaboratory.com/

- Advanced Cholesterol Profile
- Spectracell http://www.spectracell.com/
  - CardioMetabolic Profile (includes adiponectin)
- ZRT Lab http://www.zrtlab.com/
  - Weight Management Profile

Websites

Autoimmune Paleo Resources

- Autoimmune Paleo http://autoimmune-paleo.com/
  Recipes and blog on AIP
- Phoenix Helix http://www.phoenixhelix.com/
  Podcast, recipes, and blog
- The Paleo Mom http://thepaleomom.com
  Blog and recipes

BBT Charting and Monitoring Supplies

- Fairhaven Health – Fertility Monitoring Supplies http://fairhavenhealth.com
- Fertility Friend BBT Charting APP http://fertilityfriend.com
- Kindara BBT Charting APP http://kindara.com
- Ovacue Fertility Monitor http://www.ovacue.com/
- Ovagraph BBT Charting APP http://www.ovagraph.com
- Ovusense Fertility Monitor http:// Ovusense.com

Breastfeeding

- http://www.kellymom.com, blog with articles on breastfeeding, tips to increase supply
- http://www.lli.org, La Leche League—mother-to-mother breastfeeding support
- http://www.nbci.ca/, Dr. Jack Newman's wealth of information on breastfeeding including proper latch, tongue tie, and other important issues that can impact breastfeeding

Environment

- Environmental Defense Fund Seafood Selector http://seafood.edf.org
- Environmental Working Group http://www.ewg.org
  Skincare Database, Guide to Pesticides in Food, Seafood Guide, GMOs

Ketogenic Diet

- http://ketodietapp.com
- http://ruled.me

Medical Doctors Who Specialize in PCOS

- Dr. Katherine Sherif http://hospitals.jefferson.edu/find-a-doctor/s/sherif-katherine-d/
- Dr. Mark Perloe http://www.ivf.com/
- Dr. Ricardo Azziz http://people.healthsciences.ucla.edu/institution/personnel?personnel_id=75130
- Dr. Richard Legro http://www.pennstatehershey.org/web/obgyn/home
- Dr. Felice Gersh of Integrative Medical Group of Irvine http://integrativemgi.com/

Naturopathic Doctors in Your Area

- American Association of Naturopathic Physicians http://www.naturopathic.org/
- Canadian Association of Naturopathic Doctors http://www.cand.ca/

PCOS Associations

- PCOS Association http://www.pcosupport.org/
- PCOS Awareness Association http://www.pcosaa.org/
- PCOS Foundation http://www.pcosfoundation.org/
- Verity http://www.verity-pcos.org.uk/

PCOS and Hormone Health Blogs and Websites

- Hormone Soup: A website and online TV show founded by Sonya Satveit dedicated to raising consciousness around hormone issues in women. http://hormonesoup.com/

- IVF.ca: An interactive forum for patients undergoing fertility challenges and/or IVF procedures. http://ivf.ca

- PCOS Challenge: An online support network founded by Sasha Ottey dedicated to raising awareness and support for PCOS. http://www. pcoschallenge.com/

- PCOS Diet Support: A website and blog from Tarryn Bell sharing PCOS resources and nutritional information. http://www.pcosdietsupport.com/

- PCOS Diva: A website including many informative articles and expert interviews along with hollistic lifestyle programs to support women with PCOS, founded by PCOS Diva Amy Medling. http://pcosdiva.com

- PCOS Nutrition Center: A website and blog founded by dietician Angela Grassi focused on the nutritional treatment of PCOS. http:// pcosnutrition.com/

- SoulCysters: An interactive forum including resources for women with PCOS. http://soulcysters.com/

NOTES

Chapter 1

1   Boyle, Jacqueline, and Helena J. Teede. 2016. "Polycystic Ovary Syndrome: An Update." *Australian Family Physician* 41 (10): 752-56. http://www.racgp.org.au/afp/2012/october/polycystic-ovary-syndrome/.

2   Lujan, Marla E., Brittany Y. Jarrett, Eric D. Brooks, Jonathan K. Reines, Andrew K. Peppin, Narry Muhn, Ehsan Haider, Roger A. Pierson, and Donna R. Chizen. 2013. "Updated Ultrasound Criteria for Polycystic Ovary Syndrome: Reliable Thresholds for Elevated Follicle Population and Ovarian Volume." *Human Reproduction* 28 (5): 1361-68. doi:10.1093/humrep/det062.

3   Guastella, Ettore, Rosa Alba Longo, and Enrico Carmina. 2010. "Clinical and Endocrine Characteristics of the Main Polycystic Ovary Syndrome Phenotypes." *Fertility and Sterility* 94 (6): 2197-2201. doi:10.1016/j.fertnstert.2010.02.014.

4   Shroff, Rupal, Craig H. Syrop, William Davis, Bradley J. Van Voorhis, and Anuja Dokras. 2007. "Risk of Metabolic Complications in the New PCOS Phenotypes Based on the Rotterdam Criteria." *Fertility and Sterility* 88 (5): 1389-95. doi:10.1016/j.fertnstert.2007.01.032.

5   Livadas, Sarantis, and Evanthia Diamanti-Kandarakis. 2013. "Polycystic Ovary Syndrome: Definitions, Phenotypes and Diagnostic Approach." *Frontiers of Hormone Research* 40: 1-21. doi:10.1159/000341673.

6   Jamil, Avin S., Shahla K. Alalaf, Namir G. Al-Tawil, and Talha Al-Shawaf. 2016. "Comparison of Clinical and Hormonal Characteristics among Four Phenotypes of Polycystic Ovary Syndrome Based on the Rotterdam Criteria." *Archives of Gynecology and Obstetrics* 293 (2): 447-56. doi:10.1007/s00404-015-3889-5.

Chapter 2

1   González, Frank. 2012. "Inflammation in Polycystic Ovary Syndrome: Underpinning of Insulin Resistance and Ovarian Dysfunction." *Steroids* 77 (4): 300-305. doi:10.1016/j.steroids.2011.12.003.

2   Bell, Kirstine. 2014. "Clinical Application of the Food Insulin Index to Diabetes Mellitus." PhD diss., University of Sydney, School of Molecular and Microbial Bioscience. http://ses.library.usyd.edu.au:80/handle/2123/11945.

3   Bellanger, Sylvian, Marie-Claude Battista, and Jean-Patrice Baillargeon. 2014. "Insulin Resistance and Lipotoxicity in PCOS: Causes and Consequences." In *Polycystic Ovary Syndrome: Current and Emerging Concepts*, edited by Lubna Pal, 95–115. New York: Springer-Verlag. http://link.springer.com/chapter/10.1007%2F978-1-4614-8394-6_7.

4   Lammers, Karen M., Ruliang Lu, Julie Brownley, Bao Lu, Craig Gerard, Karen Thomas, Prasad Rallabhandi, et al. 2008. "Gliadin Induces an Increase in Intestinal Permeability and Zonulin Release by Binding to the Chemokine Receptor CXCR3." *Gastroenterology* 135 (1): 194–204.e3. doi:10.1053/j.gastro.2008.03.023.

5   Hollon, Justin, Elaine Leonard Puppa, Bruce Greenwald, Eric Goldberg, Anthony Guerrerio, and Alessio Fasano. 2015. "Effect of Gliadin on Permeability of Intestinal Biopsy Explants from Celiac Disease Patients and Patients with Non-Celiac Gluten Sensitivity." *Nutrients* 7 (3): 1565–76. doi:10.3390/nu7031565.

6   Zagotta, Ivana, Elitsa Y. Dimova, Jan-Bernd Funcke, Martin Wabitsch, Thomas Kietzmann, and Pamela Fischer-Posovszky. 2013. "Resveratrol Suppresses PAI-1 Gene Expression in a Human In Vitro Model of Inflamed Adipose Tissue." *Oxidative Medicine and Cellular Longevity* 2013. doi:10.1155/2013/793525.

7   Ferguson, Jane F., Claire K. Mulvey, Parth N. Patel, Rhia Y. Shah, Julia Doveikis, Weiyu Zhang, Jennifer Tabita-Martinez, et al. 2014. "Omega-3 PUFA Supplementation and the Response to Evoked Endotoxemia in Healthy Volunteers." *Molecular Nutrition & Food Research* 58 (3): 601–13. doi:10.1002/mnfr.201300368.

8   Fan, Bin, Sai-Hong Dun, Jian-Qiu Gu, Yang Guo, and Shoichiro Ikuyama. 2015. "Pycnogenol Attenuates the Release of Proinflammatory Cytokines and Expression of Perilipin 2 in Lipopolysaccharide-Stimulated Microglia in Part via Inhibition of NF-κB and AP-1 Activation." *PloS One* 10 (9). doi:10.1371/journal.pone.0137837.

9   Irandoost, Pardis, Mehrangiz Ebrahimi-Mameghani, and Saeed Pirouzpanah. 2013. "Does Grape Seed Oil Improve Inflammation and Insulin Resistance in Overweight or Obese Women?" *International Journal of Food Sciences and Nutrition* 64 (6): 706–10. doi: 10.3109/09637486.2013.775228.

10 Byun, Jae-Kyeong, Bo-Young Yoon, Joo-Yeon Jhun, Hye-Joa Oh, Eun-kyoung Kim, Jun-Ki Min, and Mi-La Cho. "Epigallocatechin-3-Gallate Ameliorates Both Obesity and Autoinflammatory Arthritis Aggravated by Obesity by Altering the Balance among CD4+ T-Cell Subsets." *Immunology Letters* 157 (1-2): 51–59. doi:10.1016/j. imlet.2013.11.006.

11 Müller, Silke, Reinhard März, Manfred Schmolz, Bernd Drewelow, Klaus Eschmann, and Peter Meiser. 2013. "Placebo-Controlled Randomized Clinical Trial on the Immunomodulating Activities of Low- and High-Dose Bromelain after Oral Administration: New Evidence on the Antiinflammatory Mode of Action of Bromelain." *Phytotherapy Research* 27 (2): 199–204. doi:10.1002/ptr.4678.

12 Lasram, Mohamed Montassar, Ines Bini Dhouib, Alya Annabi, Saloua El Fazaa, and Najoua Gharbi. 2015. "A Review on the Possible Molecular Mechanism of Action of N-acetylcysteine against Insulin Resistance and Type-2 Diabetes Development." *Clinical Biochemistry* 48 (16-17): 1200–1208. doi:10.1016/j.clinbiochem.2015.04.017.

13 Naz, Rajesh K. 2011. "Can Curcumin Provide an Ideal Contraceptive?" *Molecular Reproduction and Development* 78 (2): 116–23. doi:10.1002/mrd.21276.

14 Khajehdehi, Parviz, Batol Zanjaninejad, Elham Aflaki, Mohamadali Nazarinia, Fariborz Azad, Leila Malekmakan, and Gholam-Reza Dehghanzadeh. 2012. "Oral Supplementation of Turmeric Decreases Proteinuria, Hematuria, and Systolic Blood Pressure in Patients Suffering from Relapsing or Refractory Lupus Nephritis: A Randomized and Placebo-Controlled Study." *Journal of Renal Nutrition* 22 (1): 50–57. doi:10.1053/j.jrn.2011.03.002.

15 Ghosh, Shatadal, Sharmistha Banerjee, and Parames C Sil. 2015. "The Beneficial Role of Curcumin on Inflammation, Diabetes and Neurodegenerative Disease: A Recent Update." *Food and Chemical Toxicology: An International Journal Published for the British Industrial Biological Research Association* 83: 111–24. doi:10.1016/j.fct.2015.05.022.

16 López, Patricia, Miguel Gueimonde, Abelardo Margolles, and Ana Suárez. 2010. "Distinct Bifidobacterium Strains Drive Different Immune Responses in Vitro." *International Journal of Food Microbiology* 138 (1-2): 157–65. doi:10.1016/j. ijfoodmicro.2009.12.023.

17 Wang, Xuexuan, Mary Carmen Valenzano, Joanna M. Mercado, E. Peter Zurbach, and James M. Mullin. 2013. "Zinc Supplementation Modifies Tight Junctions and Alters Barrier Function of CACO-2 Human Intestinal Epithelial Layers." *Digestive Diseases and Sciences* 58 (1): 77–87. doi:10.1007/s10620-012-2328-8.

Chapter 3

1 Carmina, Enrico. 2013. "Obesity, Adipokines and Metabolic Syndrome in Polycystic Ovary Syndrome." *Frontiers of Hormone Research* 40 (January): 40–50. doi:10.1159/000341840.

2 Altuntas, Yuksel, Muammer Bilir, Sema Ucak, and Sadi Gundogdu. 2005. "Reactive Hypoglycemia in Lean Young Women with PCOS and Correlations with Insulin Sensitivity and with Beta Cell Function." *European Journal of Obstetrics, Gynecology, and Reproductive Biology* 119 (2): 198–205. doi:10.1016/j.ejogrb.2004.07.038.

3 Tomiyama, A. Janet, Jeffrey M. Hunger, Jolene Nguyen-Cuu, Christine Wells. 2016. "Misclassification of Cardiometabolic Health When Using Body Mass Index Categories in NHANES 2005–2012." *International Journal of Obesity* February 2016. doi: 10.1038/ ijo.2016.17

4 Greenwood, E.A., L.A. Pasch, K. Shinkai, M.I. Cedars, and H.G. Huddleston. 2014. "The Power of Sweat: Vigorous Exercise Is Associated with Improved Outcomes in Polycystic Ovarian Syndrome (PCOS) Independent of Total Exercise Volume." *Fertility and Sterility* 102 (3): e38. doi:10.1016/j.fertnstert.2014.07.137.

5 Lee, Heetae, and GwangPyo Ko. 2014. "Effect of Metformin on Metabolic Improvement and Gut Microbiota." *Applied and Environmental Microbiology* 80 (19): 5935–43. doi:10.1128/AEM.01357-14.

6 Corominas-Faja, Bruna, Rosa Quirantes-Piné, Cristina Oliveras-Ferraros, Alejandro Vazquez-Martin, Sílvia Cufí, Begoña Martin-Castillo, Vicente Micol, Jorge Joven, Antonio Segura-Carretero, and Javier A. Menendez. 2012. "Metabolomic Fingerprint Reveals That Metformin Impairs One-Carbon Metabolism in a Manner Similar to the Antifolate Class of Chemotherapy Drugs." *Aging* 4 (7): 480–98. http://www.pubmedcentral.nih.gov/articlerender. fcgi?artid=3433934&tool=pmcentrez&rendertype=abstract.

7   Lisi, Franco, Piero Carfagna, Mario Montanino Oliva, Rocco Rago, Rosella Lisi, Roberta Poverini, Claudio Manna, Elena Vaquero, Donatella Caserta, Valeria Raparelli, Roberto Marci, and Massimo Moscarini. 2012. "Pretreatment with Myo-Inositol in Non Polycystic Ovary Syndrome Patients Undergoing Multiple Follicular Stimulation for IVF: A Pilot Study." *Reproductive Biology Endocrinology* 10 (52). doi: 10.1186/1477-7827-10-52.

8   Baillargeion, Jean-Patrice, Evanthia Diamanti-Kandarakis, Richard E. Ostlund, J R, Teimuraz Apridonidze, Maria J. Iuorno, and John E. Nestler. 2006. "Altered D-Chiro-Inositol Urinary Clearance in Women with Polycystic Ovary Syndrome." *Diabetes Care* 29 (2). doi: 10.2337/diacare.29.02.dco5-1070.

9   Zhang, Xu, Yufeng Zhao, Jia Xu, Zhengsheng Xue, Menghui Zhang, Xiaoyan Pang, Xiaojun Zhang, and Liping Zhao. 2015. "Modulation of Gut Microbiota by Berberine and Metformin during the Treatment of High-Fat Diet-Induced Obesity in Rats." *Scientific Reports* 5 (September): 14405. doi:10.1038/srep14405.

10   Wei, Wei, Hongmin Zhao, Aili Wang, Ming Sui, Kun Liang, Haiyun Deng, Yukun Ma, Yajuan Zhang, Hongxiu Zhang, and Yuanyuan Guan. 2011. "A Clinical Study on the Short-Term Effect of Berberine in Comparison to Metformin on the Metabolic Characteristics of Women with Polycystic Ovary Syndrome." *European Journal of Endocrinology* 166 (1): 99–105. doi:10.1530/EJE-11-0616.

11   Ortega, Israel, and Antoni J. Duleba. 2015. "Ovarian Actions of Resveratrol." *Annals of the New York Academy of Sciences* 1348: 86–96. doi:10.1111/nyas.12875.

12   Benrick, Anna, Manuel Maliqueo, Sun Miao, Jesus A. Villanueva, Yi Feng, Claes Ohlsson, Antoni J. Duleba, and Elisabet Stener-Victorin. 2013. "Resveratrol Is Not as Effective as Physical Exercise for Improving Reproductive and Metabolic Functions in Rats with Dihydrotestosterone-Induced Polycystic Ovary Syndrome." *Evidence-Based Complementary and Alternative Medicine* 2013: doi:10.1155/2013/964070.

13   McCarty, Mark F. 2002. "Glucomannan Minimizes the Postprandial Insulin Surge: A Potential Adjuvant for Hepatothermic Therapy." *Medical Hypotheses* 58 (6): 487–90. http://www.ncbi.nlm.nih.gov/pubmed/12323114.

14   Montagut, Gemma, Cinta Bladé, Mayte Blay, Juan Fernández-Larrea, Gerard Pujadas, M. Josepa Salvadó, Lluís Arola, Montserrat Pinent, and Anna Ardévol. 2010. "Effects of a Grapeseed Procyanidin Extract (GSPE) on Insulin Resistance." *The Journal of Nutritional Biochemistry* 21 (10): 961–67. doi:10.1016/j.jnutbio.2009.08.001.

15   Jamilian, Mehri, Maryamalsadat Razavi, Zohreh Fakhrie Kashan, Yasser Ghandi, Tayebeh Bagherian, and Zatollah Asemi. 2015. "Metabolic Response to Selenium Supplementation in Women with Polycystic Ovary Syndrome: A Randomized, Double-Blind, Placebo-Controlled Trial." *Clinical Endocrinology* 82 (6): 885–91. doi:10.1111/cen.12699.

16   Masharani, Umesh, Christine Gjerde, Joseph L. Evans, Jack F. Youngren, and Ira D. Goldfine. 2010. "Effects of Controlled-Release Alpha Lipoic Acid in Lean, Nondiabetic Patients with Polycystic Ovary Syndrome." *Journal of Diabetes Science and Technology* 4 (2): 359–64. http://www.pubmedcentral.nih.gov/articlerender.fcgi?artid=2864173&tool=pmcentrez&rendertype=abstract.

17 Kort, Daniel H., and Roger A. Lobo. 2014. "Preliminary Evidence That Cinnamon Improves Menstrual Cyclicity in Women with Polycystic Ovary Syndrome: A Randomized Controlled Trial." *American Journal of Obstetrics and Gynecology* 211 (5): 487.e1–487.e6. doi:10.1016/j.ajog.2014.05.009.

18 Hassanzadeh Bashtian, Maryam, Seyed Ahmad Emami, Nezhat Mousavifar, Habib Allah Esmaily, Mahmoud Mahmoudi, and Amir Hooshang Mohammad Poor. 2013. "Evaluation of Fenugreek (Trigonella foenum-graceum L.), Effects Seeds Extract on Insulin Resistance in Women with Polycystic Ovarian Syndrome." *Iranian Journal of Pharmaceutical Research* 12 (2): 475–81. http://www.pubmedcentral.nih.gov/articlerender.fcgi?artid=3813238&tool=pmcentrez&rendertype=abstract.

Chapter 4

1 Lerchbaum, Elisabeth, Verena Schwetz, Albrecht Giuliani, Thomas Pieber, and Barbara Obermayer-Pietsch. 2012. "Opposing Effects of Dehydroepiandrosterone Sulfate and Free Testosterone on Metabolic Phenotype in Women with Polycystic Ovary Syndrome." *Fertility and Sterility* 98 (5): 1318–25.e1. doi: 10.1016/j.fertnstert.2012.07.1057.

2 Tsilchorozidou, Tasoula, John W. Honour, and Gerard S. Conway. 2003. "Altered Cortisol Metabolism in Polycystic Ovary Syndrome: Insulin Enhances 5alpha-Reduction but Not the Elevated Adrenal Steroid Production Rates." *The Journal of Clinical Endocrinology and Metabolism* 88 (12): 5907–13. doi:10.1210/jc.2003-030240.

3 Plat, Laurence, Maria M. Byrne, Jeppe Sturis, Kenneth S. Polonsky, Jean Mockel, Françoise Féry, and Eve Van Cauter. 1996. "Effects of Morning Cortisol Elevation on Insulin Secretion and Glucose Regulation in Humans." *The American Journal of Physiology* 270 (1 Pt 1): E36–42. http://www.ncbi.nlm.nih.gov/pubmed/8772471.

4 Weiner, Cindy L., Margaret Primeau, and David A. Ehrmann. 2004. "Androgens and Mood Dysfunction in Women: Comparison of Women With Polycystic Ovarian Syndrome to Healthy Controls." *Psychosomatic Medicine* 66 (3): 356–62. doi:10.1097/01. psy.0000127871.46309.fe.

5 Dokras, Anuja. 2012. "Mood and Anxiety Disorders in Women with PCOS." *Steroids* 77 (4): 338–41. doi:10.1016/j.steroids.2011.12.008.

6 Delarue, Jacques, Oscar Matzinger, Christophe Binnert, Philippe Schneiter, Rene Chioléro, and Luc Tappy. 2003. "Fish Oil Prevents the Adrenal Activation Elicited by Mental Stress in Healthy Men." *Diabetes & Metabolism* 29 (3): 289–95. http://www.ncbi. nlm.nih.gov/pubmed/12909818.

7 Unno, Keiko, Kazuaki Iguchi, Naoki Tanida, Keisuke Fujitani, Nina Takamori, Hiroyuki Yamamoto, Naoto Ishii, et al. 2013. "Ingestion of Theanine, an Amino Acid in Tea, Suppresses Psychosocial Stress in Mice." *Experimental Physiology* 98 (1): 290–303. doi:10.1113/expphysiol.2012.065532.

8 Hellhammer, Juliane, Dominic Vogt, Nadin Franz, Ulla Freitas, and David Rutenberg. 2014. "A Soy-Based Phosphatidylserine/ Phosphatidic Acid Complex (PAS) Normalizes the Stress Reactivity of Hypothalamus-Pituitary-Adrenal-Axis in Chronically Stressed Male Subjects: A Randomized, Placebo-Controlled Study." *Lipids in Health and Disease* 13: 121. doi:10.1186/1476-511X-13-121.

9   Monteleone, Palmiero, Mario Maj, Lucia Beinat, Mariantonietta Natale, Dargut Kemali, "Blunting by Chronic Phosphatidylserine Administration of the Stress-Induced Activation of the Hypothalamo-Pituitary-Adrenal Axis in Healthy Men." *European Journal of Clinical Pharmacology* 42 (4): 385-8

10   Armanini, Decio, Mee Jung Mattarello, Cristina Fiore, Guglielmo Bonanni, Carla Scaroni, Paola Sartorato, and Mario Palermo. "Licorice Reduces Serum Testosterone in Healthy Women." *Steroids* 69 (11-12): 763–66. doi:10.1016/j.steroids.2004.09.005.

11   Yu, Jin, Dongxia Zhai, Li Hao, Danying Zhang, Lingling Bai, Zailong Cai, and Chaoqin Yu. 2014. "Cryptotanshinone Reverses Reproductive and Metabolic Disturbances in PCOS Model Rats via Regulating the Expression of CYP17 and AR." *Evidence-Based Complementary and Alternative Medicine* 2014. doi:10.1155/2014/670743.

12   Grundman, Oliver, Yuanhua Lv, Olaf Kelber, Veronika Butterweck. 2010. "Mechanism of St. John's Wort Extract (STW3-VI) During Chronic Restraint Stress Is Mediated by the Interrelationship of the Immune, Oxidative Defense, and Neuroendocrine System." *Neuropharmacology* 58 (4–5): 767-73. http://www.ncbi.nlm.nih.gov/pubmed/20036263?itool=EntrezSystem2.PEntrez.Pubmed.Pubmed_ResultsPanel.Pubmed_RVDocSum&ordinalpos=2.

13   Yang, Shui-Jin, Hai-Yang Yu, Dan-Yu Kang, Zhan-Qiang Ma, Rong Hui Qu, Qiang Fu, Shi_Ping Ma. 2014. "Antidepressant-like Effects of Salidroside on Olfactory Bulbectomy-Induced Pro-Inflammatory Cytokine Production and Hyperactivity of HPA Axis in Rats." Pharmacology Biochemistry and Behavior Sept (124): 451–7. doi: 10.1016/j.pbb.2014.07.015.

14   Panossian, Alexander, Marina Hambardzumyan, Areg Hovhanissyan, and Georg Wikman. 2007. "The Adaptogens Rhodiola and Schizandra Modify the Response to Immobilization Stress in Rabbits by Suppressing the Increase of Phosphorylated Stress-Activated Protein Kinase, Nitric Oxide, and Cortisol." *Drug Target Insights* 2: 39–54.

15   Held, Katja, Irina A. Antonijevic, Heike E. Kunzel, Manfred Uhr, Thomas C. Wetter, I. C. Golly, A. Steiger, and Harald Murck. 2002. "Oral Mg (2+) Supplementation Reverses Age-Related Neuroendocrine and Sleep EEG Changes in Humans." *Pharmacopsychiatry* 35 (4): 135–43. doi: 10.1055/s-2002-33195.

16   Infante, Jose R., Fernando Peran, Margarita Martinez, Ana Roldan, Rafael Poyatos, Concha Ruiz, Francisco Samaniego, and Frederico Garrido. 1998. "ACTH and Beta-Endorphin in Transcendental Meditation." *Physiological Behavior* 64 (3): 311–315.

17   Stefanaki, Charikleia, Flora Bacopoulou, Sarantis Livadas, Anna Kandaraki, Athanasios Karachalios, George P. Chrousos, and Evanthia Kandarakis. 2015. "Impact of a Mindfulness Stress Management Program on Stress Anxiety, Depression, and Quality of Life in Women with Polycystic Ovary Syndrome: A Randomized Controlled Trial." *Stress* 18 (1): 57_66. doi: 10.3109/10253890.2014.974030.

18   Manincor, Michael de, Alan Bensoussan, Caroline Smith, Paul Fahey, and Suzanne Bourchier. "Establishing Key Components of Yoga Interventions for Reducing Depression and Anxiety, and Improving Well-Being: A Delphi Method Study." *2015. BMC Complementary and Alternative Medicine.* 15: 85. doi: 10.1186/s12906-015-0614-7.

19   Rofey, Dana L., Eva M. Szigethy, Robert B. Noll, Ronald E. Dahl, Emily Lobst, and Silva A. Arslanian. 2009. "Cognitive-Behavioral Therapy for Physical and Emotional Disturbances in Adolescents with Polycystic Ovary Syndrome: A Pilot Study." *Journal of Pediatric Psychology* 34 (2): 156–63. doi:10.1093/jpepsy/jsn057.

Chapter 5

1 Gersh, Felice. 2015. *Anti-Aging Therapeutics Volume XVII, Volume 17, Volume 12.* Chicago: A4M American Academy of Anti-Aging Medicine. https://books.google.com/books?id=xY3oCgAAQBAJ&pgis=1.

2 Hillman, Kathrin and Ulrike Blume-Peytavi. 2009. "Diagnosis of Hair Disorders." *Seminars in Cutaneous Medicine and Surgery* 28 (1): 19–32.

3 Hacivelioglu, Servet, Ayse Nur Cakir Gungor, Meryem Gencer, Ahmet Uysal, Deniz Hizli, Evrim Koc, Emine Cosar. 2013. "Acne Severity and the Global Acne Grading System in Polycystic Ovary Syndrome." *International Journal of Gynecology & Obstetrics* 123 (1): 33_36. doi:10.1016/j.ijgo.2013.05.005

4 Adeniji, Anthonia Adinike, P. A. Essah, J. E. Nestler, K I Cheang. 2016. "Metabolic Effects of a Commonly Used Combined Hormonal Oral Contraceptive in Women with and without Polycystic Ovary Syndrome." *Journal of Women's Health.* www.ncbi.nlm.nih.gov/pubmed/26871978.

5 Somjen, Dalia, Esther Knoll, Jacob Vaya, Naftali Stern, and Snait Tamir. 2004. "Estrogen-like Activity of Licorice Root Constituents: Glabridin and Glabrene, in Vascular Tissues in Vitro and in Vivo." *The Journal of Steroid Biochemistry and Molecular Biology* 91 (3): 147–55. doi:10.1016/j.jsbmb.2004.04.003.

6 Tamir, S., M. Eizenberg, D. Somjen, S. Izrael, and J. Vaya. 2001. "Estrogen-Like Activity of Glabrene and Other Constituents Isolated from Licorice Root." *The Journal of Steroid Biochemistry and Molecular Biology* 78 (3): 291–98. http://www.ncbi.nlm.nih.gov/pubmed/11595510.

7 Takeuchi, Toru, Osamu Nishii, Takashi Okamura, and Tsutomu Yaginuma. 1991. "Effect of Paeoniflorin, Glycyrrhizin, and Glycyrrhetic Acid on Ovarian Androgen Production." *The American Journal of Chinese Medicine* 19 (1): 73–78. doi:10.1142/S0192415X91000119.

8 Hiipakka, Richard A., Han-Zhong Zhang, Wei Dai, Qing Dai, and Shutsung Liao. 2002. "Structure-Activity Relationships for Inhibition of Human 5alpha-Reductases by Polyphenols." *Biochemical Pharmacology* 63 (6): 1165–76. http://www.ncbi.nlm.nih.gov/pubmed/11931850.

9 Nagata, Chisato, Michinori Kabuto, and Hiroyuki Shimizu. 1998. "Association of Coffee, Green Tea, and Caffeine Intakes with Serum Concentrations of Estradiol and Sex Hormone-Binding Globulin in Premenopausal Japanese Women." *Nutrition and Cancer* 30 (1): 21–24. doi:10.1080/01635589809514635.

10 Fujita, Rumi, Jie Liu, Kuniyoshi Shimizu, Fumiko Konishi, Kiyoshi Noda, Shoichiro Kumamoto, Chie Ueda, et al. 2005. "Anti-Androgenic Activities of Ganoderma Lucidum." *Journal of Ethnopharmacology* 102 (1): 107–12. doi:10.1016/j.jep.2005.05.041.

11 Liu, Jie, Kuniyoshi Shimizu, Fumiko Konishi, Kiyoshi Noda, Shoichiro Kumamoto, Kenji Kurashiki, and Ryuichiro Kondo. 2007. "Anti-Androgenic Activities of the Triterpenoids Fraction of Ganoderma Lucidum." *Food Chemistry* 100 (4): 1691–96. doi:10.1016/j.foodchem.2006.01.003.

12 Akdoğan, Mehmet, Mehmet Numan Tamer, Erkan Cüre, Medine Cumhur Cüre, Banu Kale Köroğlu, and Namik Delibaş. 2007. "Effect of Spearmint (Mentha spicata Labiatae) Teas on Androgen Levels in Women with Hirsutism." *Phytotherapy Research* 21 (5): 444–47. doi:10.1002/ptr.2074.

13 Grant, Paul. 2010. "Spearmint Herbal Tea Has Significant Anti-Androgen Effects in Polycystic Ovarian Syndrome. A Randomized Controlled Trial." *Phytotherapy Research* 24 (2): 186–88. doi:10.1002/ptr.2900.

14 Prager, Nelson, Karen Bickett, Nita French, and Geno Marcovici. 2004. "A Randomized, Double-Blind, Placebo-Controlled Trial to Determine the Effectiveness of Botanically Derived Inhibitors of 5-Alpha-Reductase in the Treatment of Androgenetic Alopecia." *Journal of Alternative and Complementary Medicine* 8 (2): 143–52. doi:10.1089/107555302317371433.

15 Murata, Kazuya, Kazuma Noguchi, Masato Kondo, Mariko Onishi, Naoko Watanabe, Katsumasa Okamura, and Hideaki Matsuda. 2013. "Promotion of Hair Growth by *Rosmarinus officinalis* Leaf Extract." *Phytotherapy Research* 27 (2): 212–17. doi:10.1002/ptr.4712.

16 Fischer, Tobias, G Burmeister, H W Schmidt, and Peter Elsner. 2004. "Melatonin Increases Anagen Hair Rate in Women with Androgenetic Alopecia or Diffuse Alopecia: Results of a Pilot Randomized Controlled Trial." *British Journal of Dermatology* 150 (2): 341-5. doi: 10.1111/j.1365-2133.2004.05685.x

17 Hostanska, Katarina, Thomas Nisslein, Johannes Freudenstein, Juergen Reichling, and Reinhard Saller. "Apoptosis of Human Prostate Androgen-Dependent and -Independent Carcinoma Cells Induced by an Isopropanolic Extract of Black Cohosh Involves Degradation of Cytokeratin (CK) 18." *Anticancer Research* 25 (1A): 139–47. http://www.ncbi.nlm.nih.gov/pubmed/15816531.

18 Seidlová-Wuttke, D., L. Pitzel, P. Thelen, and W. Wuttke. 2006. "Inhibition of 5α-Reductase in the Rat Prostate by Cimicifuga Racemosa." *Maturitas* 55: S75–82. doi:10.1016/j.maturitas.2006.06.019.

19 Rushton, D. Hugh, M. J. Norris, R. Dover, and Nina Busuttil. 2002. "Causes of Hair Loss and the Developments in Hair Rejuvenation." *International Journal of Cosmetic Science* 24 (1): 17–23. doi:10.1046/j.0412-5463.2001.00110.x.

20 Rushton, D. Hugh, and Isobel D. Ramsay. 1992. "The Importance of Adequate Serum Ferritin Levels During Oral Cyproterone Acetate and Ethinyl Oestradiol Treatment of Diffuse AndroDen-Dependent Alopecia in Women." *Clinical Endocrinology* 36 (4): 421–27. http://www.ncbi.nlm.nih.gov/pubmed/1424176.

21 Darabi R., Hafezi M.A., Akbarloo N. 2007. "A Comparative, Investigator-Blind Study of Topical Tea Tree Oil versus Erythromycin Gel in the Treatment of Acne." *European Society of Clinical Microbiology and Infectious Diseases* 15. http://www.blackwellpublishing.com/eccmid15/abstract.asp?id=36262.

22 Bassett, I. B., D. L. Pannowitz, Ross St C. Barnetson. 1990. "A Comparative Study of Tea Tree Oil vs. Benzoylperoxide in the Treatment of Acne." *The Medical Journal of Australia* 153 (8): 455–58

23 Kwon, Hyuck Hoon, Ji Young Yoon, Seon Yong Park, Seonguk Min, and Dae Hun Suh. 2014. "Comparison of Clinical and Histological Effects between Lactobacillus-Fermented Chamaecyparis Obtusa and Tea Tree Oil for the Treatment of Acne: An Eight-Week Double-Blind Randomized Controlled Split-Face Study." *Dermatology (Basel, Switzerland)* 229 (2). 102–9. doi:10.1159/000362491.

Chapter 6

1   Bhide, Priya, Merve Dilgil, Anil Gudi, Amit Shah, Charity Akwaa, and Roy Homburg. 2015. "Each Small Antral Follicle in Ovaries of Women with Polycystic Ovary Syndrome Produces More Antimüllerian Hormone than Its Counterpart in a Normal Ovary: An Observational Cross-Sectional Study." *Fertility and Sterility* 103 (2): 537–41. doi:10.1016/j.fertnstert.2014.10.033.

2   Cimino, Irene, Filippo Casoni, Xinhuai Liu, Andrea Messina, Jyoti Parkash, Soazik. 2016. "Novel Role for Anti-Mullerian Hormone in the Regulation of GnRH Neuron Excitability and Hormone Secretion." *Nature Communications* 7:10055. doi: 10.1038/ncomms10055.

3   Ong, Kee J., Efstathios Theodoru, and William Ledger. 2006. "Long-Term Consequence of Polycystic Ovarian Syndrome." *Current Obstetrics & Gynaecology* 16 (6): 333–36. doi:10.1016/j.curobgyn.2006.09.002.

4   Takahashi, K., and M. Kitao. "Effect of TJ-68 (shakuyaku-kanzo-to) on Polycystic Ovarian Disease." *International Journal of Fertility and Menopausal Studies* 39 (2): 69–76. http://www.ncbi.nlm.nih.gov/pubmed/8012442.

5   Düker, E. M., L. Kopanski, H. Jarry, and W. Wuttke. 1991. "Effects of Extracts from Cimicifuga racemosa on Gonadotropin Release in Menopausal Women and Ovariectomized Rats." *Planta Medica* 57 (5): 420–24. doi:10.1055/s-2006-960139.

6   Shahin, Ahmed Y, Alaa M. Ismail, Kamal M. Zahran, and Ahmad M. Makhlouf. 2008. "Adding Phytoestrogens to Clomiphene Induction in Unexplained Infertility Patients—a Randomized Trial." *Reproductive Biomedicine Online* 16 (4): 580–88. http://www.ncbi.nlm.nih.gov/pubmed/18413068.

7   Shahin, Ahmed Y, and Safwat A Mohammed. 2014. "Adding the Phytoestrogen Cimicifugae Racemosae to Clomiphene Induction Cycles with Timed Intercourse in Polycystic Ovary Syndrome Improves Cycle Outcomes and Pregnancy Rates—a Randomized Trial." *Gynecological Endocrinology* 30 (7): 505–10. doi:10.3109/09513590.2014.895983.

8   Ye, Qi, Qiao-yan Zhang, Cheng-jian Zheng, Yang Wang, and Lu-ping Qin. 2010. "Casticin, a Flavonoid Isolated from Vitex rotundifolia, Inhibits Prolactin Release in Vivo and in Vitro." *Acta Pharmacologica Sinica* 31 (12): 1564–68. doi:10.1038/aps.2010.178.

9   Nasri, Sima, Shahrbano Oryan, Ali Haeri Rohani, and Gholam Reza Amin. 2007. "The Effects of Vitex Agnus Castus Extract and Its Interaction with Dopaminergic System on LH and Testosterone in Male Mice." *Pakistan Journal of Biological Sciences* 10 (14): 2300–2307. http://www.ncbi.nlm.nih.gov/pubmed/19070148.

10 Ibrahim, N. A., A. S. Shalaby, R. S. Farag, G. S. Elbaroty, S. M. Nofal, and E. M. Hassan. 2008. "Gynecological Efficacy and Chemical Investigation of Vitex Agnus-Castus L. Fruits Growing in Egypt." *Natural Product Research* 22 (6): 537–46. doi:10.1080/14786410701592612.

11 Webster, D. E., J. Lu, S. N. Chen, N. R. Farnsworth, and Z. Jim Wang. 2006. "Activation of the Mu-Opiate Receptor by Vitex agnus-castus Methanol Extracts: Implication for Its Use in PMS." *Journal of Ethnopharmacology* 106 (2): 216–21. doi:10.1016/j.jep.2005.12.025.

12   Samochowiec L, Glaesmer R, Samochowiec J. 2005. "No TEinfluss von Monchspfeffer Auf Die Konzentration von Beta-Endorphine Im Serum Weiblicher Ratten. Aerztezeitschrift Fur Naturheilverfahrenitle." *SOFW-Journal* 131: 1–4.

13   Silberstein, S. D., and G. R. Merriam. 2000. "Physiology of the Menstrual Cycle." *Cephalalgia* 20 (3). 148–54. doi:10.1046/j.1468-2982.2000.00034.x.

14   Pasqualotto, Eleonora B., Fabio Firmbach Pasqualotto, Bernardo P. Sobreiro, and Antonio Marmo Lucon. 2005. "Female Sexual Dysfunction: The Important Points to Remember." *Clinics (São Paulo, Brazil)* 60 (1): 51–60. doi:/S1807-59322005000100011. (REV et al. 2007; Pasqualotto et al. 2005).

15   Zangeneh, Farideh Zafari, A. Mohammadi, Sh Ejtemaeimehr, Mohammad Mahdi Naghizadeh, and Aminee Fatemeh. 2011. "The Role of Opioid System and Its Interaction with Sympathetic Nervous System in the Processing of Polycystic Ovary Syndrome Modeling in Rat." *Archives of Gynecology and Obstetrics* 283 (4): 885–92. doi:10.1007/s00404-010-1776-7.

Chapter 7

1   Mueller, A, Schofl, R Dittrich, S Cupisti, P G Oppelt, R L Schild, M W Beckmann, L Haberle. 2009. "Thyroid-Stimulating Hormone Is Associated with Insulin Resistance Independently of Body Mass Index and Age in Women with Polycystic Ovary Syndrome." *Human Reproduction* 24 (11): 2924–30.

2   Janssen, Onno Eilard, Nadine Mehlmauer, Susanne Hahn, Alexandra H Offner, Roland Gaertner. 2004. "High Prevelence of Autoimmune Thyroiditis in Patients with Polycystic Ovary Syndrome." *European Journal of Endocrinology 150* (3): 363–9. doi: 10.1530/eje.0.1500363.

3   NACB: Laboratory Support for the Diagnosis and Monitoring of Thyroid Disease. Laurence M. Demers, Ph.D., F.A.C.B.and Carole A. Spencer Ph.D., F.A.C.B. (page 175)

4   Mueller, A, Schofl, R Dittrich, S Cupisti, P G Oppelt, R L Schild, M W Beckmann, L Haberle. 2009. "Thyroid-Stimulating Hormone Is Associated with Insulin Resistance Independently of Body Mass Index and Age in Women with Polycystic Ovary Syndrome." *Human Reproduction* 24 (11): 2924–30.

5   Dittrich. R., N. Kajaia, S. Cupisti, I. Hoffmann, M. W. Beckmann, A. Mueller. 2009. "Association of Thyroid-Stimulating Hormone with Insulin Resistance and Androgen Paramneters in Women with PCOS." *Reproductive Biomedicine Online* 19 (3)L: 319–25.

6   Selva, David M and Geoffrey L Hammond. 2009. "Thyroid Hormones Act Indirectly to Increase Sex Hormone-Binding Globulin Production by Liver via Hepatocyte Nuclear Factor-4." *Journal of Molecular Endocrinology* 43 (1): 19–27. doi: 10.1677/JME-09-0025.

7   Muderris, Iptisam Ipek, Abdullah Boztosun, Gokalp Oner, Fahri Bayram. 2011. "Effect of Thyroid Hormone Replacement Therapy on Ovarian Volume and Androgen Hormones in Patients with Untreated Primary Hypothyroidism." *Annals of Saudi Medicine* 31 (2): 145–51. doi: 10.4103/0256-4947.77500.

8   Kachuei, M., F. Jafari, A. Kachuei, A.H. Keshteli. 2011. "Prevalence of Autoimmune Thyroiditis in Patients with Polycystic Ovary Syndrome." *Archive of Gynecology and Obstetrics* 285 (3): 853–6. doi: 1007/s00404-011-2040-5.

9   Du, Dafeng and Li Xuelian. 2013. "The Relationship Between Thyroiditis and Polycystic
     Ovary Syndrome: A Meta-Analysis." *International Journal of Clinical and Experimental
     Medicine* 6 (10): 880–9. http://www.ncbi.nlm.nih.gov/pmc/articles/PMC3832324/.

10   Ott, Johannes, Stefanie Austin, Christine Kurz, Kazem Nouri, Stefan Wirth, Johannes C.
     Huber, and Klaus Mayerhofer. "Elevated Antithyroid Peroxidase Antibodies Indicating
     Hashimoto's Thyroiditis Are Associated with the Treatment Response in Infertile
     Women with Polycystic Ovary Syndrome." *Fertility and Sterility* 94 (7): 2895–2897. doi:
     10.1016/j.fertnstert.2010.05.063.

11   Kiortsis DN, Durack I, Turpin G 1999 Effects of a Low-Calorie Diet on Resting
     Metabolic Rate and Serum Triiodothyronine Levels in Obese Children. *European
     Journal of Pediatrics* 158: 446–450.

12   Arujo, Raphael L., Bruno M Andrade, Alvaro S Padron, Mandeep P Gaidhu,
     Ruby L Perry, Denise P Caralho, and Rolando B Ceddia. 2010. "High-Fat Diet
     Increases Thyrotropin and Oxygen Consumption without Altering Circulating
     3,5,3'-Triidothyronine (T3) and Thyroxine in Rats: The Role of Iodothyronine
     Deiodinases, Reverse T3 Production, and Whole-Body Fat Oxidation." *Endocrinology*
     151 (7): 3460–9. doi: 10.1210/en.2010/en.2010-0026.

13   Tripathi, Yamini B., O. P. Malhotra, and San N. Tripathi. 1984. "Thyroid Stimulating
     Action of Z-Guggulsterone Obtained from Commiphora Mukul." *Planta Medica* 50 (1):
     78–80. doi:10.1055/s-2007-969626.

Chapter 8

1   Akin, Leyla, Mustafa Kendirci, Figen Narin, Selim Kurtoglu, Recep Saraymen, and
     Meda Kondolot. 2014. "The Endocrine Disruptor Bisphenol A May Play a Role in the
     Aetiopathogenesis of Polycystic Ovary Syndrome in Adolescent Girls." *Acta Paediatrica*
     104 (4). doi: 10.1111/apa.12885

2   Tarantino, Giovanni, Rossella Valentino, Carolina D. Somma, Vittoria D'Esposito,
     Federica Passaretti, Genoveffa Pizza, Valentina Brancato, Francesco Orio, Pietro
     Formisano, Annamaria Colao, and Silvia Savastano. 2012. "Bisphenol A in Polycystic
     Ovary Syndrome and Its Association with Liver-Spleen Axis." *Clinical Endocrinology* 78
     (3). doi: 10.1111/j.1365-2265.2012.04500.x

3   Nilsson, Eric, Ginger Larsen, Mohan Manikkam, Carlos Guerrero-Bosagna, Marina
     I. Savenkova, and Michael K. Skinner. 2012. "Environmentally Induced Epigenetic
     Transgenerational Inheritance of Ovarian Disease." *PLOS ONE* 7 (5): e36129. doi:
     10.1371/journal.pone.0036129.

4   Vargas-Mendoza, Nancy, Eduardo Madrigal-Santillán, Angel Morales-González, Jaime
     Esquivel-Soto, Cesar Esquivel-Chirino, Manuel García-Luna Y. González-Rubio, Juan
     A. Gayosso-de-Lucio, and José A. Morales-González. 2014. "Hepatoprotective Effect of
     Silymarin." *World Journal of Hepatology* 6 (3): 144–49. doi:10.4254/wjh.v6.i3.144.

5   Dinkova-Kostova, A. T., and P. Talalay. 1999. "Relation of Structure of Curcumin
     Analogs to Their Potencies as Inducers of Phase 2 Detoxification Enzymes."
     Carcinogenesis 20 (5): 911–14. http://www.ncbi.nlm.nih.gov/pubmed/10334211.

6   Lin, H. J., N. M. Probst-Hensch, A. D. Louie, I. H. Kau, J. S. Witte, S. A. Ingles, H. D. Frankl, E. R. Lee, and R. W. Haile. 1998. "Glutathione Transferase Null Genotype, Broccoli, and Lower Prevalence of Colorectal Adenomas." *Cancer Epidemiology, Biomarkers & Prevention* 7 (8): 647–52. http://www.ncbi.nlm.nih.gov/pubmed/9718215.

7   Kensler, T. W., T. J. Curphey, Y. Maxiutenko, and B. D. Roebuck. 2000. "Chemoprotection by Organosulfur Inducers of Phase 2 Enzymes: Dithiolethiones and Dithiins." *Drug Metabolism and Drug Interactions* 17 (1-4): 3–22. http://www.ncbi.nlm.nih.gov/pubmed/11201301.

Chapter 9

1   Holt, S. H., J. C. Miller, and P. Petocz. 1997. "An Insulin Index of Foods: The Insulin Demand Generated by 1000-kJ Portions of Common Foods." *American Journal of Clinical Nutrition* 66 (5): 1264–76. http://ajcn.nutrition.org/content/66/5/1264.abstract.

2   Bao, Jiansong, Fiona Atkinson, Peter Petocz, Walter C. Willett, and Jennie C. Brand-Miller. 2011. "Prediction of Postprandial Glycemia and Insulinemia in Lean, Young, Healthy Adults: Glycemic Load Compared with Carbohydrate Content Alone." *The American Journal of Clinical Nutrition* 93 (5): 984–96. doi:10.3945/ajcn.110.005033.

3   ewg. 2003. "PCBs in Farmed Salmon." Accessed February 12, 2016. http://www.ewg.org/research/pcbs-farmed-salmon.

4   Handa, Y., H. Fujita, S. Honma, H. Minakami, and R. Kishi. 2009. "Estrogen Concentrations in Beef and Human Hormone-Dependent Cancers." *Annals of Oncology* 20 (9): 1610–11. doi:10.1093/annonc/mdp381.

5   Daley, Cynthia A., Amber Abbott, Patrick S. Doyle, Glenn A. Nader, and Stephanie Larson. 2010. "A Review of Fatty Acid Profiles and Antioxidant Content in Grass-Fed and Grain-Fed Beef." *Nutrition Journal* 9 (1). doi:10.1186/1475-2891-9-10.

6   Ponnampalam, Eric N., Neil J. Mann, and Andrew J. Sinclair. 2006. "Effect of Feeding Systems on Omega-3 Fatty Acids, Conjugated Linoleic Acid and Trans Fatty Acids in Australian Beef Cuts: Potential Impact on Human Health." *Asia Pacific Journal of Clinical Nutrition* 15 (1): 21–29. http://www.ncbi.nlm.nih.gov/pubmed/16500874.

7   Giovannucci, E. "Nutrition, Insulin, Insulin-like Growth Factors and Cancer." *Hormone and Metabolic Research* 35 (11-12): 694–704. doi:10.1055/s-2004-814147.

8   Blum, Jürg W., and Craig R. Baumrucker. 2008. "Insulin-like Growth Factors (IGFs), IGF Binding Proteins, and Other Endocrine Factors in Milk: Role in the Newborn." *Advances in Experimental Medicine and Biology* 606: 397–422. doi:10.1007/978-0-387-74087-4_16.

9   Tian, Xiaodong, Kun Hao, Changfu Qin, Kun Xie, Xuehai Xie, and Yinmo Yang. 2013. "Insulin-Like Growth Factor 1 Receptor Promotes the Growth and Chemoresistance of Pancreatic Cancer." *Digestive Diseases and Sciences* 58 (9): 2705–12. doi:10.1007/s10620-013-2673-2.

10 Loglisci, Ralph. 2010. "New FDA Numbers Reveal Food Animals Consume Lion's Share of Antibiotics." *Center for a Livable Future (blog)* December 23. http://www.livablefutureblog.com/2010/12/new-fda-numbers-reveal-food-animals-consume-lion%E2%80%99s-share-of-antibiotics.

11 Madjd, Ameneh, Moira A. Taylor, Alireza Delavari, Reza Malekzadeh, Ian A. Macdonald, and Hamid R. Farshchi. 2015. "Effects on Weight Loss in Adults of Replacing Diet Beverages with Water during a Hypoenergetic Diet: A Randomized, 24-Wk Clinical Trial." *The American Journal of Clinical Nutrition* 102 (6): 1305–12. doi:10.3945/ajcn.115.109397.

12 Ritchie, K., I. Carrière, A. de Mendonca, F. Portet, J. F. Dartigues, O. Rouaud, P. Barberger-Gateau, and M. L. Ancelin. 2007. "The Neuroprotective Effects of Caffeine: A Prospective Population Study (the Three City Study)." *Neurology* 69 (6): 536–45. doi:10.1212/01.wnl.0000266670.35219.0c.

13 Takami, Hidenobu, Mariko Nakamoto, Hirokazu Uemura, Sakurako Katsuura, Miwa Yamaguchi, Mineyoshi Hiyoshi, Fusakazu Sawachika, Tomoya Juta, and Kokichi Arisawa. 2013. "Inverse Correlation Between Coffee Consumption and Prevalence of Metabolic Syndrome: Baseline Survey of the Japan Multi-Institutional Collaborative Cohort (J-MICC) Study in Tokushima, Japan." *Journal of Epidemiology* 23 (1): 12–20. doi:10.2188/jea.JE20120053.

14 González, Frank, Chang Ling Sia, Marguerite K. Shepard, Neal S. Rote, and Judi Minium. 2014. "The Altered Mononuclear Cell-Derived Cytokine Response to Glucose Ingestion Is Not Regulated by Excess Adiposity in Polycystic Ovary Syndrome." *The Journal of Clinical Endocrinology and Metabolism* 99 (11): E2244–51. doi:10.1210/jc.2014-2046.

15 Teff, Karen L., Sharon S. Elliott, Matthias Tschöp, Timothy J. Kieffer, Daniel Rader, Mark Heiman, Raymond R. Townsend, Nancy L. Keim, David D'Alessio, and Peter J. Havel. 2004. "Dietary Fructose Reduces Circulating Insulin and Leptin, Attenuates Postprandial Suppression of Ghrelin, and Increases Triglycerides in Women." *The Journal of Clinical Endocrinology and Metabolism* 89 (6): 2963–72. doi:10.1210/jc.2003-031855.

16 Turnbaugh, Peter J., Vanessa K. Ridaura, Jeremiah J. Faith, Federico E. Rey, Rob Knight, and Jeffrey I. Gordon. 2009. "The Effect of Diet on the Human Gut Microbiome: A Metagenomic Analysis in Humanized Gnotobiotic Mice." *Science Translational Medicine* 1 (6): 6ra14. doi:10.1126/scitranslmed.3000322.

17 Alang, N., and C. R. Kelly. 2015. "Weight Gain After Fecal Microbiota Transplantation." *Open Forum Infectious Diseases* 2 (1): 001-002. doi:10.1093/ofid/ofv004.

18 Fowler, Sharon P., Ken Williams, Roy G. Resendez, Kelly J. Hunt, Helen P. Hazuda, and Michael P. Stern. 2008. "Fueling the Obesity Epidemic? Artificially Sweetened Beverage Use and Long-Term Weight Gain." *Obesity* (Silver Spring, Md.) 16 (8): 1894–1900. doi:10.1038/oby.2008.284.

19 Preedy, Victor R. 2015. *Calcium: Chemistry, Analysis, Function and Effects*. Cambridge, UK: Royal Society of Chemistry. https://books.google.com/books?id=OajHCgAAQBAJ&pgis=1.

20 Feskanich, D., W. C. Willett, M. J. Stampfer, and G. A. Colditz. 1997. "Milk, Dietary Calcium, and Bone Fractures in Women: A 12-Year Prospective Study." *American Journal of Public Health* 87 (6): 992–97. doi:10.2105/AJPH.87.6.992.

21 Hollon, Justin, Elaine Leonard Puppa, Bruce Greenwald, Eric Goldberg, Anthony Guerrerio, and Alessio Fasano. 2015. "Effect of Gliadin on Permeability of Intestinal Biopsy Explants from Celiac Disease Patients and Patients with Non-Celiac Gluten Sensitivity." *Nutrients* 7 (3): 1565–76. doi:10.3390/nu7031565.

22 Lammers, Karen M., Ruliang Lu, Julie Brownley, Bao Lu, Craig Gerard, Karen Thomas, Prasad Rallabhandi, et al. 2008. "Gliadin Induces an Increase in Intestinal Permeability and Zonulin Release by Binding to the Chemokine Receptor CXCR3." *Gastroenterology* 135 (1): 194–204.e3. doi:10.1053/j.gastro.2008.03.023.

23 Jönsson, Tommy, Ashfaque A. Memon, Kristina Sundquist, Jan Sundquist, Stefan Olsson, Amarnadh Nalla, Mikael Bauer, and Sara Linse. 2015. "Digested Wheat Gluten Inhibits Binding between Leptin and Its Receptor." *BMC Biochemistry* 16: 3. doi:10.1186/s12858-015-0032-y.

24 Bray, Molly, J-Y Tsai, Carlina Villegas-Montoya, Brandon B. Boland, Zackary Blasier, Oluwaseun Egbejimi. 2005. "Timf-of-Day-Dependent Dietary FatConsumption Influences Multiple Cardiometabolic Syndrome Parameters in Mice." *International Journal of Obesity* 34 (11): 158–98.doi: 10.1038/ijo.2010.63

Appendix A

1 Biljan, M. M., R. Hemmings, and N. Brassard. 2005. "The Outcome of 150 Babies Following the Treatment with Letrozole or Letrozole and Gonadotropins." *Fertility and Sterility* 84 (Suppl 1): S95. doi: 10.1016/j.fertnstert.2005.07.230.

2 Tulandi, T., J. Martin, R. Al-Fadhli, N. Kabli, R Forman, J. Hitkari, C Librach, E Greenblatt, and R F Casper. "Congenital Malformations Among 911 Newborns Conceived After Infertility Treatment with Letrozole or Clomiphene Citrate." *Fertility and Sterility* 85 (6): 1761–5. http://www.ncbi.nlm.nih.gov/pubmed/16650422.

3 Papaleo, E., V. Unfer, J. P. Baillargeon, and T. T. Chiu. 2009. "Contribution of Myo-Inositol to Reproduction." *European Journal of Obstetrics, Gynecology, and Reproductive Biology* 147 (2): 120–23. doi:10.1016/j.ejogrb.2009.09.008.

4 Nordio, M., and E. Proietti. 2012. "The Combined Therapy with Myo-Inositol and D-Chiro-Inositol Reduces the Risk of Metabolic Disease in PCOS Overweight Patients Compared to Myo-Inositol Supplementation Alone." *European Review for Medical and Pharmacological Sciences* 16 (5): 575–81. http://www.ncbi.nlm.nih.gov/pubmed/22774396.

5 Lisi, Franco, Piero Carfagna, Mario Montanino Oliva, Rocco Rago, Rosella Lisi, Roberta Poverini, Claudio Manna, et al. 2012. "Pretreatment with Myo-Inositol in Non Polycystic Ovary Syndrome Patients Undergoing Multiple Follicular Stimulation for IVF: A Pilot Study." *Reproductive Biology and Endocrinology* 10: 52. doi:10.1186/1477-7827-10-52.

6 Isabella, Rosalbino, and Emanuela Raffone. 2012. "Does Ovary Need D-Chiro-Inositol?" *Journal of Ovarian Research* 5 (1): 14. doi:10.1186/1757-2215-5-14.

7 Woo, Irene, Kyle Tobler, Ayatallah Khafagy, Mindy S. Christianson, Melissa Yates, and Jairo Garcia. 2015. "Predictive Value of Elevated LH/FSH Ratio for Ovulation Induction in Patients with Polycystic Ovary Syndrome." *The Journal of Reproductive Medicine* 60 (11-12): 495–500. http://www.ncbi.nlm.nih.gov/pubmed/26775457.

8 Saha, Lekha, Sharonjeet Kaur, and Pradip Kumar Saha. 2013. "N-Acetyl Cysteine in Clomiphene Citrate Resistant Polycystic Ovary Syndrome: A Review of Reported Outcomes." *Journal of Pharmacology & Pharmacotherapeutics* 4 (3): 187–91. doi:10.4103/0976-500X.114597.

9   Fulghesu, Anna Maria, Mario Ciampelli, Giuseppe Muzj, Chiara Belosi, Luigi Selvaggi, Gian Franco Ayala, and Antonio Lanzone. 2002. "N-Acetyl-Cysteine Treatment Improves Insulin Sensitivity in Women with Polycystic Ovary Syndrome." *Fertility and Sterility* 77 (6): 1128–35. http://www.ncbi.nlm.nih.gov/pubmed/12057717.

10 Polyzos, Nikolaos P., Ellen Anckaert, Luis Guzman, Johan Schiettecatte, Lisbet Van Landuyt, Michel Camus, Johan Smitz, and Herman Tournaye. 2014. "Vitamin D Deficiency and Pregnancy Rates in Women Undergoing Single Embryo, Blastocyst Stage, Transfer (SET) for IVF/ICSI." *Human Reproduction* 29 (9): 2032–40. doi:10.1093/humrep/deu156.

11 An, Yuan, Zhuangzhuang Sun, Yajuan Zhang, Bin Liu, Yuanyuan Guan, and Meisong Lu. 2014. "The Use of Berberine for Women with Polycystic Ovary Syndrome Undergoing IVF Treatment." *Clinical Endocrinology* 80 (3): 425–31. doi:10.1111/cen.12294.

12 Chen, Jui-Tung, Kunihiko Tominaga, Yoshiaki Sato, Hideo Anzai, and Ryo Matsuoka. 2010. "Maitake Mushroom (Grifola frondosa) Extract Induces Ovulation in Patients with Polycystic Ovary Syndrome: A Possible Monotherapy and a Combination Therapy After Failure with First-Line Clomiphene Citrate." *Journal of Alternative and Complementary Medicine* 16 (12): 1295–99. doi:10.1089/acm.2009.0696.

13 Milewicz, Andrzej, E. Gejdel, H. Sworen, K. Sienkiewicz, J. Jedrzejak, T. Teucher, and H. Schmitz. 1993. "Vitex Agnus Castus Extract in the Treatment of Luteal Phase Defects due to Latent Hyperprolactinemia. Results of a Randomized Placebo-Controlled Double-Blind Study." *Arzneimittel-Forschung* 43 (7): 752–56. http://www.ncbi.nlm.nih.gov/pubmed/8369008.

14 Kamel, Hany H. 2013. "Role of Phyto-Oestrogens in Ovulation Induction in Women with Polycystic Ovarian Syndrome." *European Journal of Obstetrics, Gynecology, and Reproductive Biology* 168 (1): 60–63. doi:10.1016/j.ejogrb.2012.12.025.

15 Shahin, Ahmed Y., and Safwat A. Mohammed. 2014. "Adding the Phytoestrogen Cimicifugae Racemosae to Clomiphene Induction Cycles with Timed Intercourse in Polycystic Ovary Syndrome Improves Cycle Outcomes and Pregnancy Rates—A Randomized Trial." *Gynecological Endocrinology* 30 (7): 505–10. doi:10.3109/09513590.2014.895983.

16 El Refaeey, Abdelaziz, Amal Selem, and Ahmed Badawy. 2014. "Combined Coenzyme Q10 and Clomiphene Citrate for Ovulation Induction in Clomiphene-Citrate-Resistant Polycystic Ovary Syndrome." *Reproductive Biomedicine Online* 29 (1): 119–24. doi:10.1016/j.rbmo.2014.03.011.

17 Sun, Wen-Shu, Atsushi Imai, Keiko Tagami, Michiyo Sugiyama, Tatsuro Furui, and Teruhiko Tamaya. 2004. "In Vitro Stimulation of Granulosa Cells by a Combination of Different Active Ingredients of Unkei-to." *The American Journal of Chinese Medicine* 32 (4): 569–78. doi:10.1142/S0192415X0400220X.

18 Jedel, Elizabeth, Fernand Labrie, Anders Odén, Göran Holm, Lars Nilsson, Per Olof Janson, Anna-Karin Lind, Claes Ohlsson, and Elisabet Stener-Victorin. 2011. "Impact of Electro-Acupuncture and Physical Exercise on Hyperandrogenism and Oligo/amenorrhea in Women with Polycystic Ovary Syndrome: A Randomized Controlled Trial." *American Journal of Physiology - Endocrinology and Metabolism* 300 (1): E37–45. doi:10.1152/ajpendo.00495.2010.

19   Leonhardt, Henrik, Mikael Hellström, Berit Gull, Anna-Karin Lind, Lars Nilsson, Per Olof Janson, and Elisabet Stener-Victorin. 2015. "Serum Anti-Müllerian Hormone and Ovarian Morphology Assessed by Magnetic Resonance Imaging in Response to Acupuncture and Exercise in Women with Polycystic Ovary Syndrome: Secondary Analyses of a Randomized Controlled Trial." *Acta Obstetricia et Gynecologica Scandinavica* 94 (3): 279–87. doi:10.1111/aogs.12571.

20   D'Anna, Rosario, V. Di Benedetto, P Rizzo, E Raffone, Maria Lieta Interdonato, F Corrado, and Antonino Di Benedetto. 2011. "Myo-Inositol May Prevent Gestational Diabetes in PCOS Women." *Gynecological Endocrinology* 28 (6): 440–2. doi: 10.3109/09513590.2011.633665.

Appendix B

1   Tehrani, Fahimeh Ramezani, Masoud Solaymani-Dodaran, Mehdi Hedayati, and Fereidoun Azizi. 2010. "Is Polycystic Ovary Syndrome an Exception for Reproductive Aging?" *Human Reproduction* 25 (7): 1775–81. doi:10.1093/humrep/deq088.

2   Shah, D., and S. Bansal. 2014. "Polycystic Ovaries: Beyond Menopause." *Climacteric* 17 (2): 109–15. doi:10.3109/13697137.2013.828687.

3   Glintborg, Dorte, Anne Pernille Hermann, and Marianne Andersen. 2013. "Bone Mineral Density and Vitamin D in PCOS and Hirsutism." *Expert Review of Endocrinology & Metabolism* 8 (5): 449–59. doi:10.1586/17446651.2013.827384.

4   Mirabi, Parvaneh, and Faraz Mojab. 2013. "The Effects of Valerian Root on Hot Flashes in Menopausal Women." *Iranian Journal of Pharmaceutical Research* 12 (1): 217–22. http://www.pubmedcentral.nih.gov/articlerender. fcgi?artid=3813196&tool=pmcentrez&rendertype=abstract.

5   Wuttke, Wolfgang, and Dana Seidlová-Wuttke. 2015. "Black Cohosh (Cimicifuga racemosa) Is a Non-Estrogenic Alternative to Hormone Replacement Therapy." *Clinical Phytoscience* 1 (1): 12. doi:10.1186/s40816-015-0013-0.

6   Knapen, Marjo H., Nadja E. Drummen, E. Smit, Cees Vermeer, and Elke Theuwissen. 2013. "Three-Year Low-Dose Menaquinone-7 Supplementation Helps Decrease Bone Loss in Healthy Postmenopausal Women." *Osteoporosis International* 24 (9): 2499–2507. doi:10.1007/s00198-013-2325-6.

7   Spector, Tim D., Mario R. Calomme, Simon H. Anderson, Gail Clement, Liisa Bevan, Nathalie Demeester, Rami Swaminathan, Ravin Jugdaohsingh, Dirk A. Vanden Berghe, and Jonathan J. Powell. 2008. "Choline-Stabilized Orthosilicic Acid Supplementation as an Adjunct to Calcium/Vitamin D3 Stimulates Markers of Bone Formation in Osteopenic Females: A Randomized, Placebo-Controlled Trial." *BMC Musculoskeletal Disorders* 9: 85. doi:10.1186/1471-2474-9-85.

Appendix C

1   Taylor, P R. 2015. "Type 2 Diabetes Reversed by Losing Fat from Pancreas." *Newcastle Academic Health Partners*, December 1. http://www.ncl.ac.uk/press/news/2015/12/ pancreasstudy/.

2   Daniilidies, A. and K. Dinas. 2009. "Long-Term Health Consequences of Polycistic Ovarian Syndrome: A Review Analysis." *Hippokratia* 13 (2): 90–92.

3   Vassilatou, E., S. Lafoyianni, Andromachi Vryonidou, D. Ioannidis, Lamprini Kosma, K. Katsoulis, E. Papavassiliou, and I. Tzavara. 2010. "Increased Androgen Bioavailability Is Associated with Non-Alcoholic Fatty Liver Disease in Women with Polycystic Ovary Syndrome." *Human Reproduction* 25 (1): 212–20. doi:10.1093/humrep/dep380.

4   Dunn, Winston, Ronghui Xu, and Jeffrey B. Schwimmer. 2008. "Modest Wine Drinking and Decreased Prevalence of Suspected Nonalcoholic Fatty Liver Disease." *Hepatology* 47 (6): 1947–54. doi:10.1002/hep.22292.

5   Lee, Gene S., Jim S. Yan, Raymond K. Ng, Sanjay Kakar, and Jacquelyn J. Maher. 2007. "Polyunsaturated Fat in the Methionine-Choline-Deficient Diet Influences Hepatic Inflammation but Not Hepatocellular Injury." *Journal of Lipid Research* 48 (8): 1885–96. doi:10.1194/jlr.M700181-JLR200.

6   Stanković, Milena N., Dušan Mladenović, Milica Ninković, Ivana Ethuričić, Slađana Sobajić, Bojan Jorgačević, Silvio de Luka, Rada Jesic Vukicevic, and Tatjana S. Radosavljević. 2014. "The Effects of α-Lipoic Acid on Liver Oxidative Stress and Free Fatty Acid Composition in Methionine-Choline Deficient Diet-Induced NAFLD." *Journal of Medicinal Food* 17 (2): 254–61. doi:10.1089/jmf.2013.0111.

7   Loguercio, Carmela, Pietro Andreone, Ciprian Brisc, Michaela Cristina Brisc, Elisabetta Bugianesi, Maria Chiaramonte, Carmela Cursaro, et al. 2012. "Silybin Combined with Phosphatidylcholine and Vitamin E in Patients with Nonalcoholic Fatty Liver Disease: A Randomized Controlled Trial." *Free Radical Biology & Medicine* 52 (9): 1658–65. doi:10.1016/j.freeradbiomed.2012.02.008.

8   Gottschau, Mathilde, Susanne Krüger Kjaer, Allan Jensen, Christian Munk, and Lene Mellemkjaer. 2015. "Risk of Cancer among Women with Polycystic Ovary Syndrome: A Danish Cohort Study." *Gynecologic Oncology* 136 (1): 99–103. doi:10.1016/j.ygyno.2014.11.012.

9   Ezzat, Shereen, Sylvia L. Asa, William T. Couldwell, Charles E. Barr, William E. Dodge, Mary Lee Vance, and Ian E. McCutcheon. 2004. "The Prevalence of Pituitary Adenomas: A Systematic Review." *Cancer* 101 (3): 613–19. doi:10.1002/cncr.20412.

INDEX

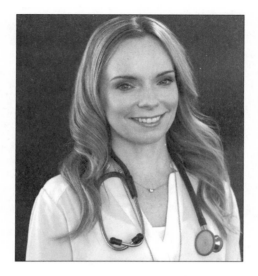

ABOUT THE AUTHOR

Dr. Fiona McCulloch has worked with thousands of people seeking better health over the past fifteen years of her practice. She is committed to health education and advocacy, empowering her patients with the most current information on health topics and natural medicine therapies with a warm, empathic approach.

Dr. Fiona has published many articles in publications for health professionals on a variety of topics including PCOS, thyroid health, autoimmunity, and infertility. Her popular research-based blog receives a monthly readership of twenty thousand per month. *8 Steps to Reverse Your PCOS* is Dr. Fiona's first book.

Dr. Fiona is a medical advisor for IVF.ca, Canada's premier fertility community, and is on the medical advisory committee for the PCOS Awareness Association. As a woman with PCOS herself, she is dedicated to increasing both awareness and research of this important condition that has far-reaching effects on the lives of so many women.

Fiona also frequently lectures to professionals, including naturopathic doctors and integrative medicine clinicians, and to students at the Canadian College of Naturopathic Medicine. Dr. Fiona is a graduate of the Canadian College of Naturopathic Medicine (2001) and the University of Guelph (biological science/molecular biology and genetics).